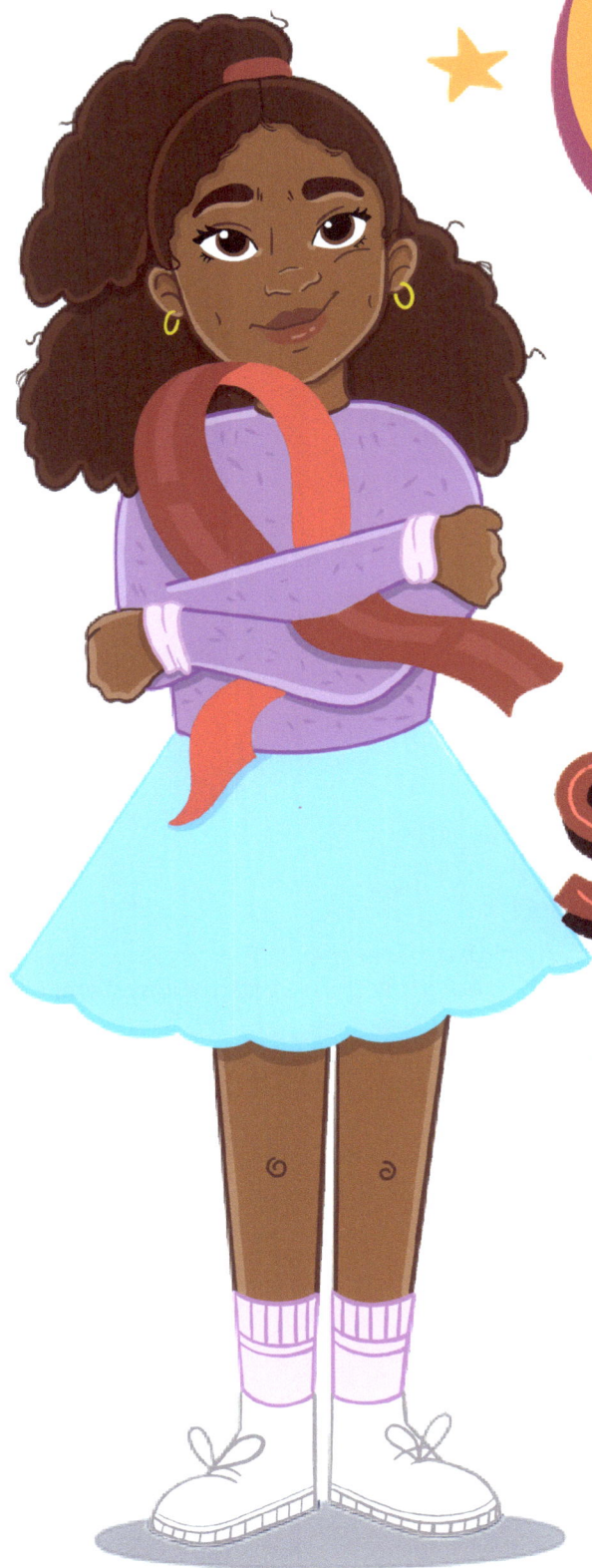

CAI'S ABC'S of SICKLE CELL

Written By Cai Stoudemire and Richon Badger

Illustrated By Barderies Hampton

ISBN 979-8-218-30820-9
Library of Congress Control Number: 2024905070
Printed in the United States of America
First Printing, 2023
Photos provided by the Badger/Stoudemire Family

Written by Cai Stoudemire and Richon Badger
Illustrated by Barderies Hampton
www.caistrong.com

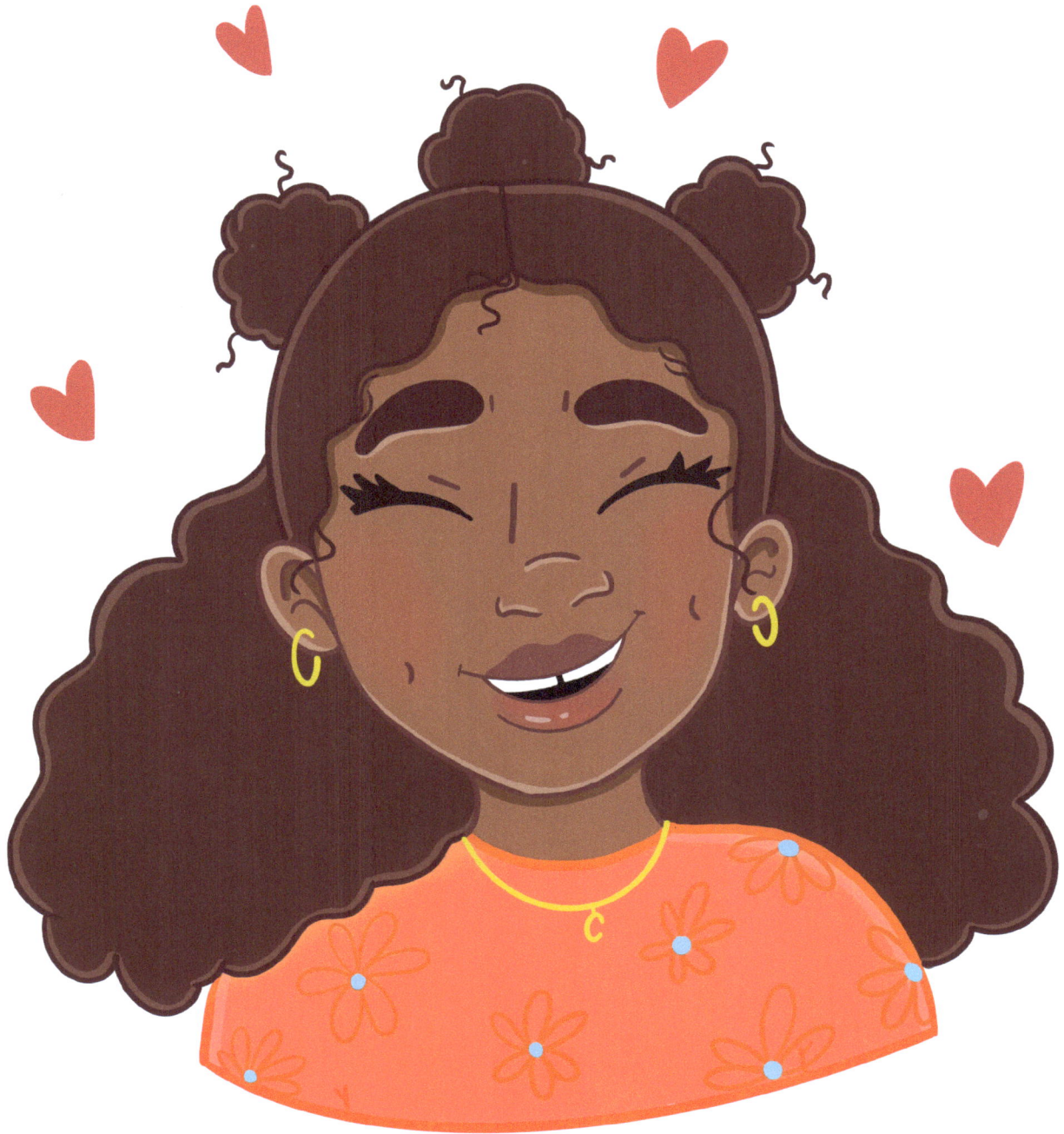

This is dedicated to Cai.
May you grow stronger,
wiser and lovelier by the day.
I love you, Mom.

WHAT IS SICKLE CELL?

Sickle Cell is a genetic blood disease that causes the red blood cells to be C or sickle shaped, instead of the normal donut shape.

A is for Acute chest syndrome. Acute chest happens when sickle cells stick together and block the flow of oxygen in tiny vessels in the lungs.

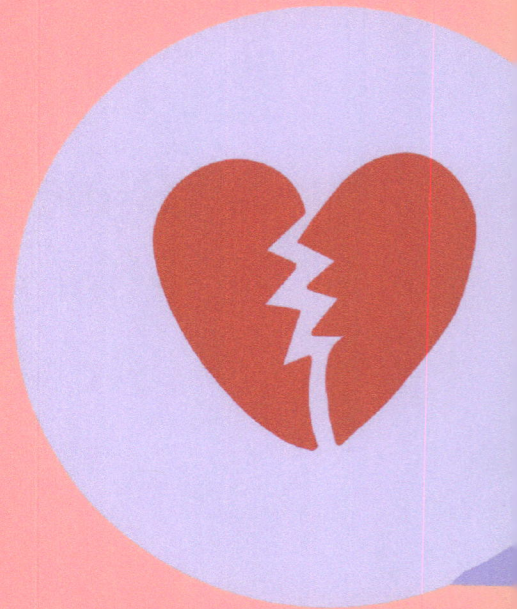

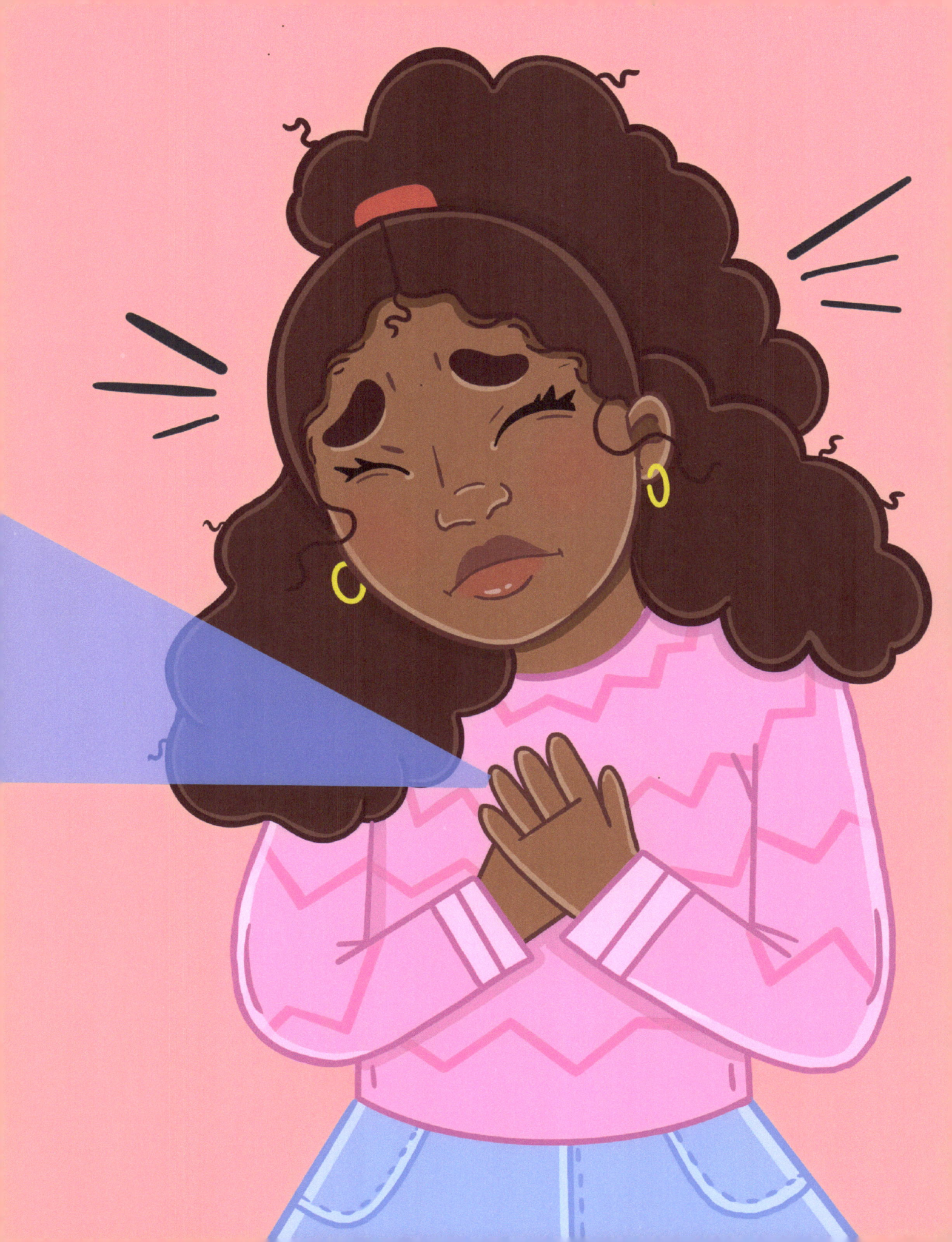

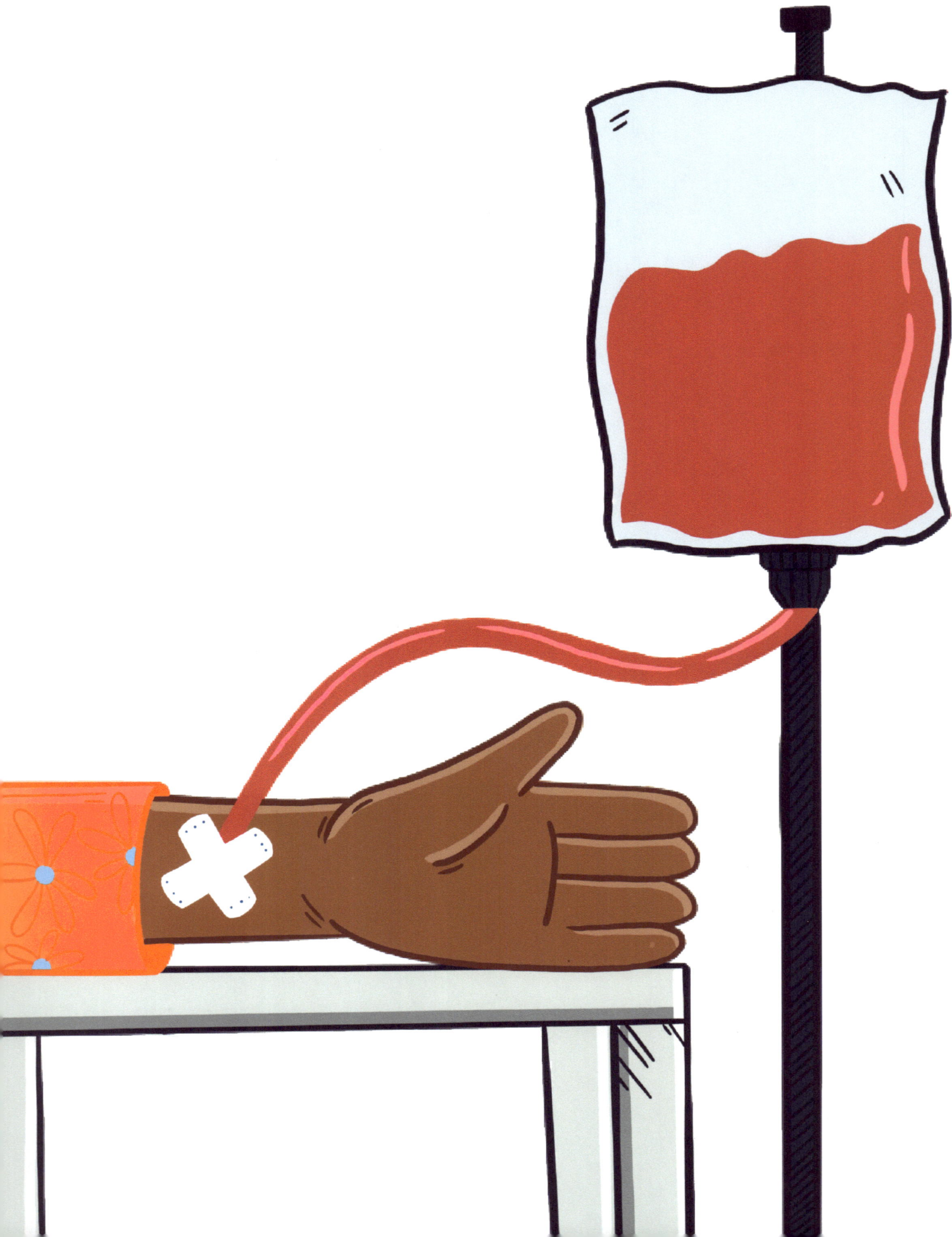

B is for Blood transfusion. Blood transfusions are used to boost the level of normal red blood cells vs sickled red blood cells in the body.

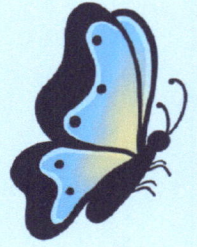

C is for Cai, of course!
I was diagnosed with Sickle Cell Beta
Zero Thalassemia and I like dogs.

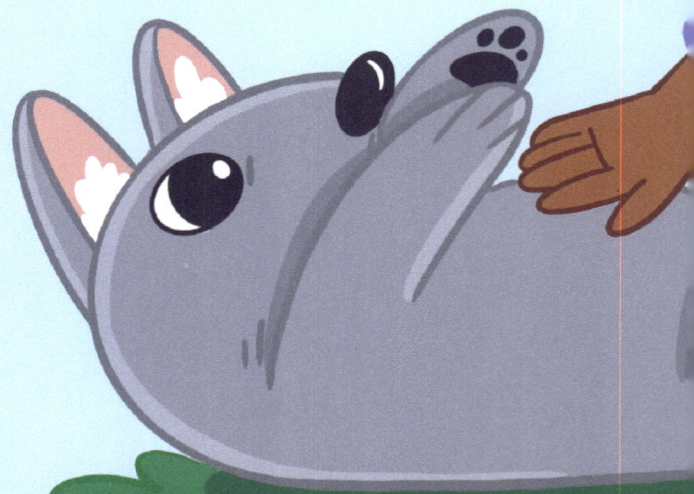

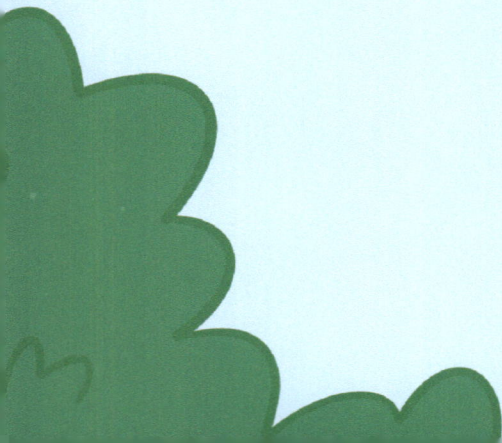

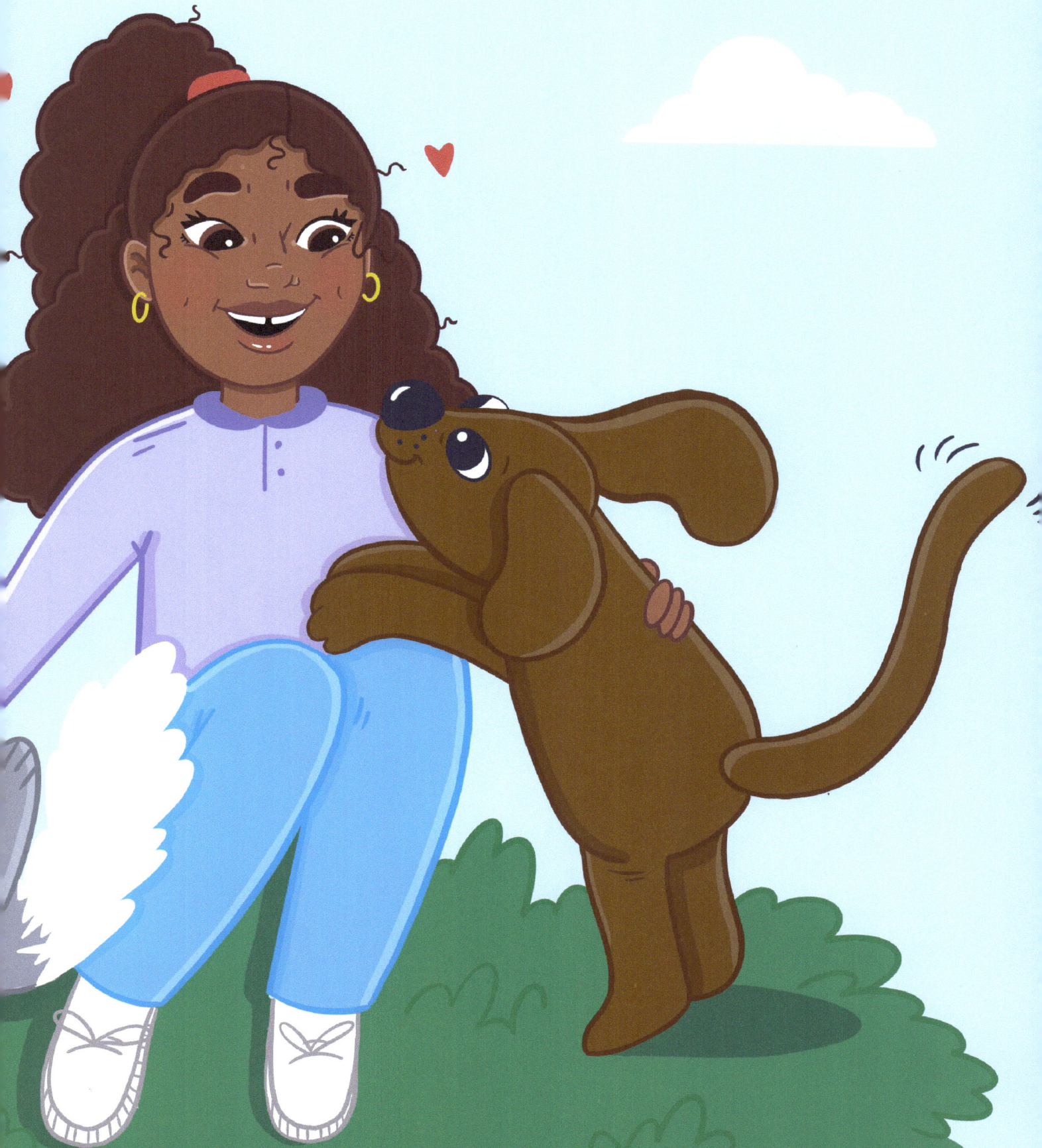

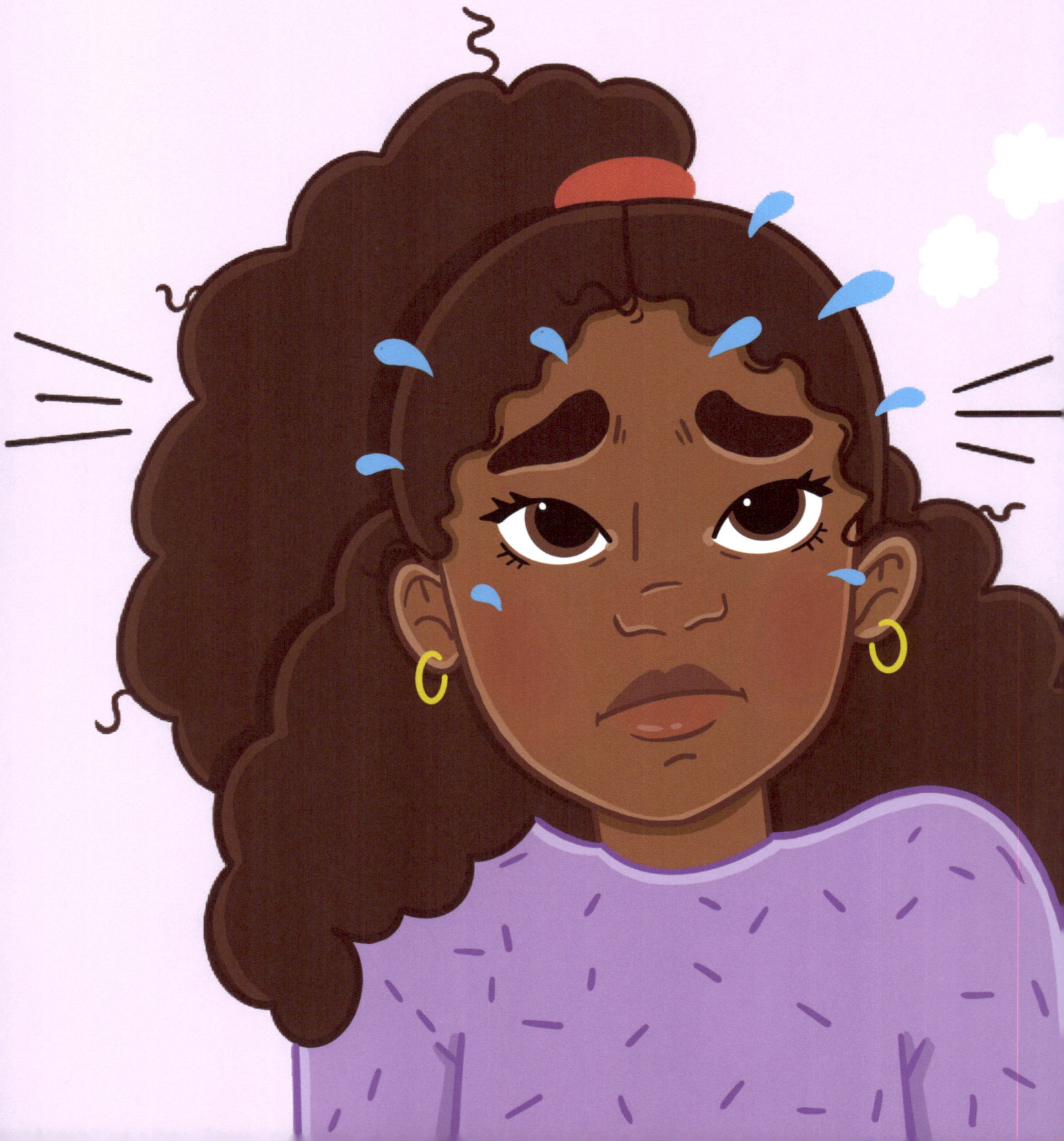

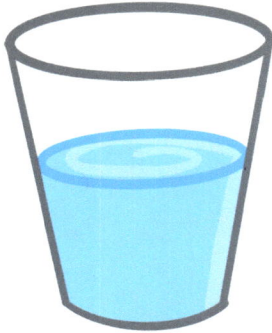

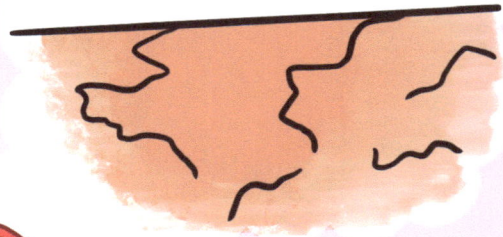

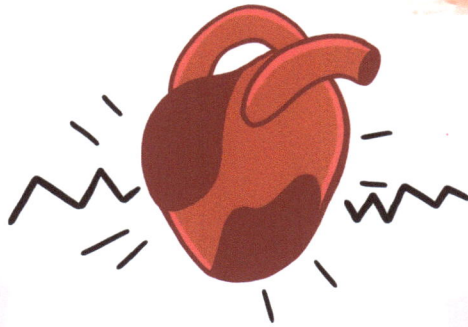

D is for Dehydration.
Dehydration can cause the red
blood cells to sickle, constantly
drinking fluids can prevent this.

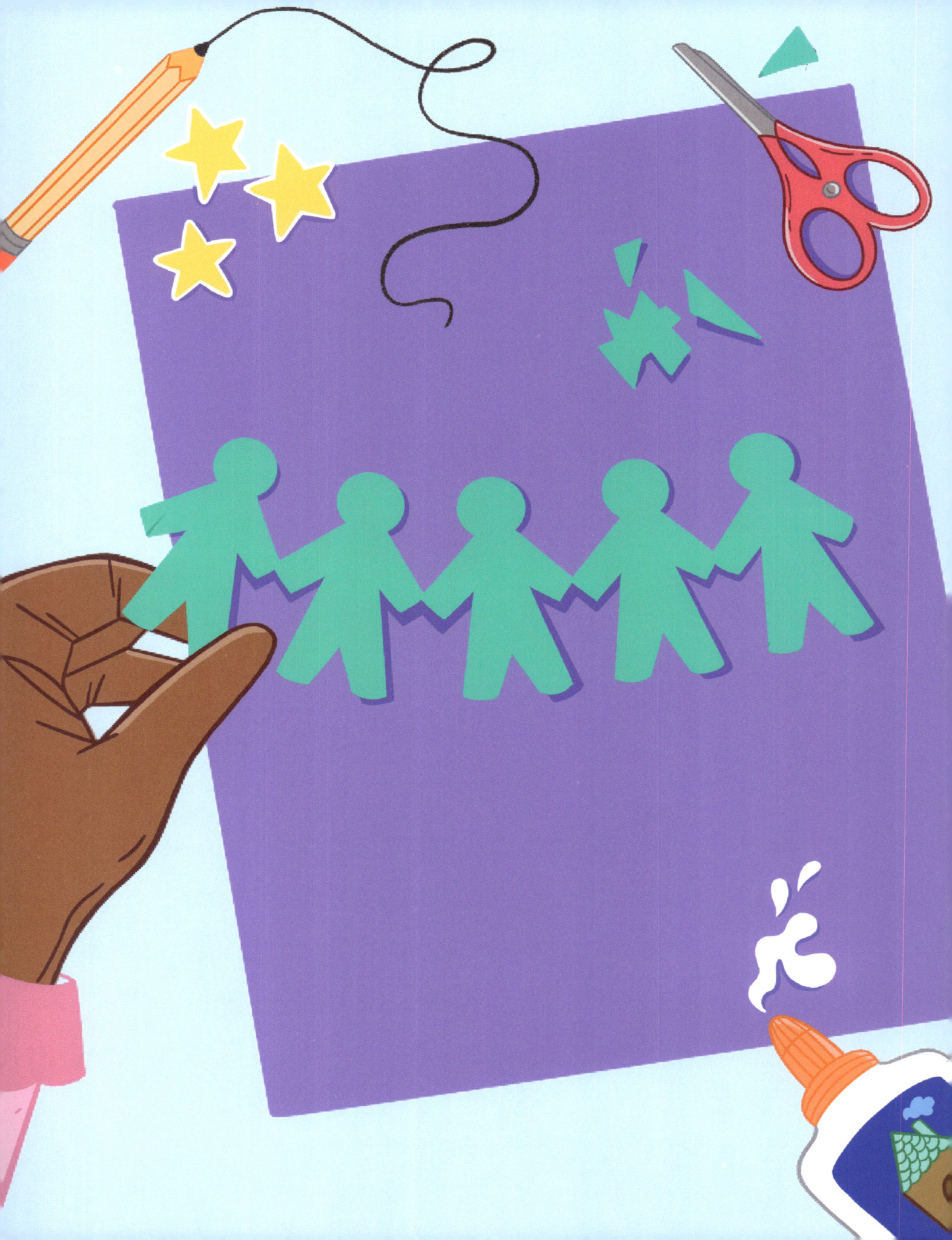

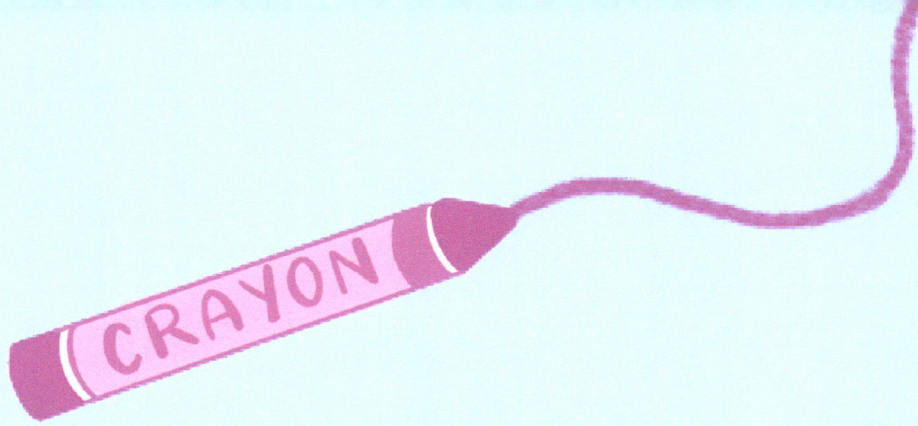

E is for Everyone.
Everyone deserves love,
joy and patience.

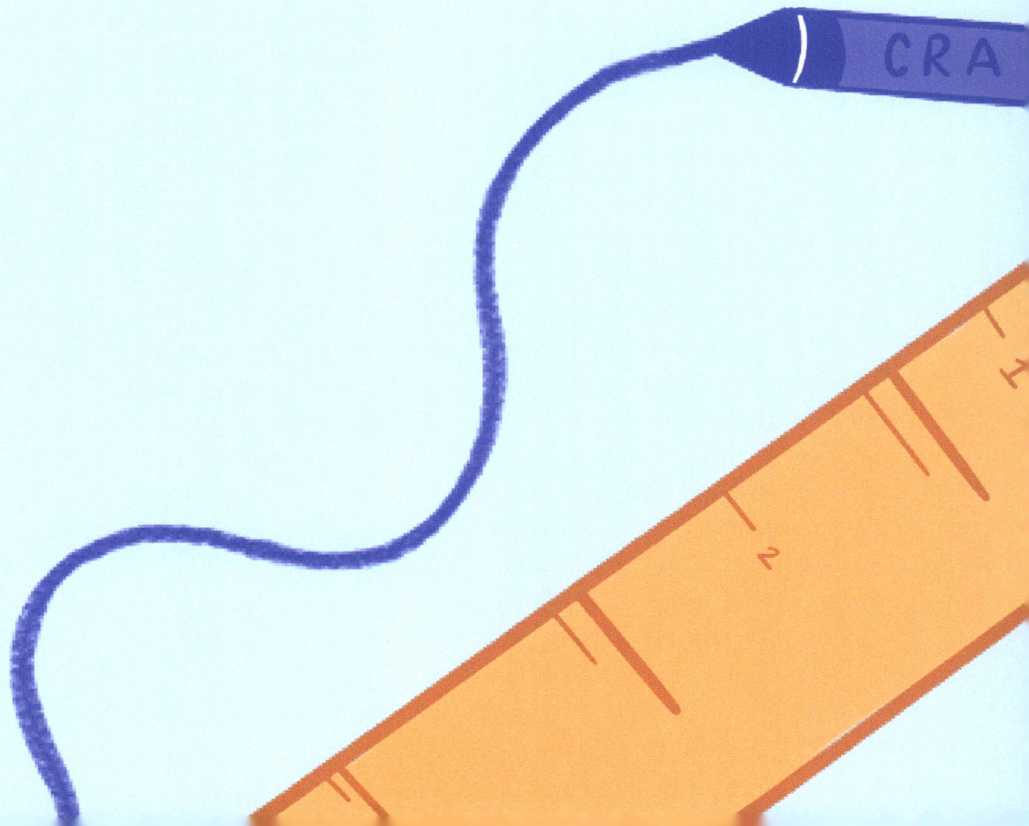

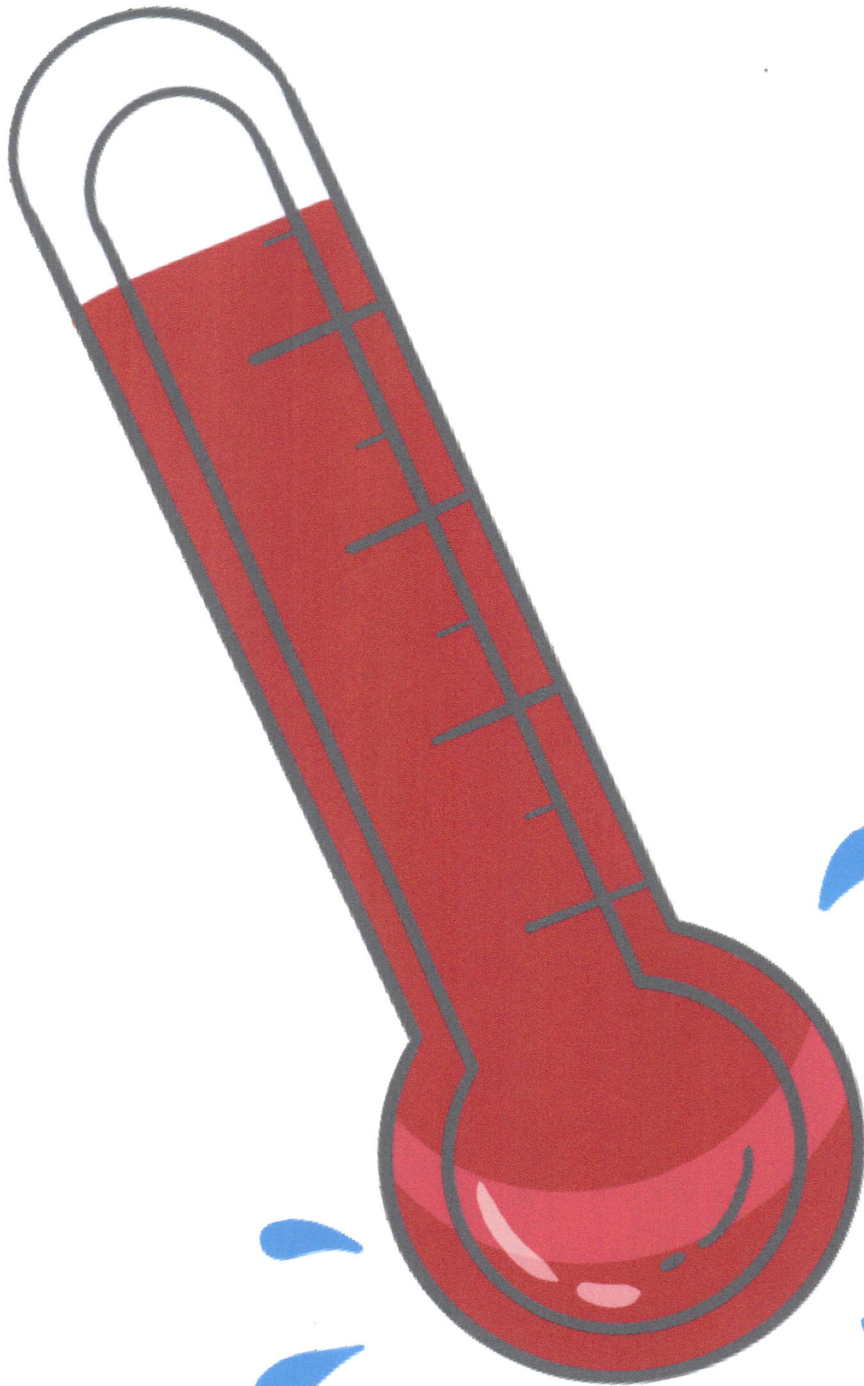

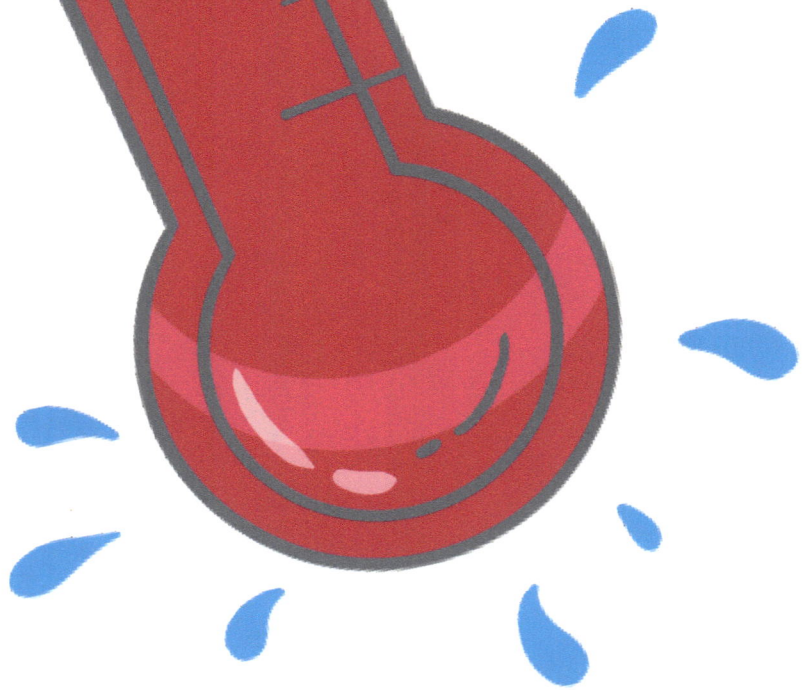

F is for Fever.
Fever is a telltale sign of sickness
or specifically Sickle Cell crisis,
especially in children who
can't verbalize their pain.
A child Sickle Cell patient, like me,
has to go to the ER whenever
a fever of 101.5 °F spikes.

G is for Gene.
Sickle Cell is a genetic disease.
It happens when one hemoglobin S gene
is passed down from one parent as well as
another abnormal hemoglobin gene from
the other parent, to the child.

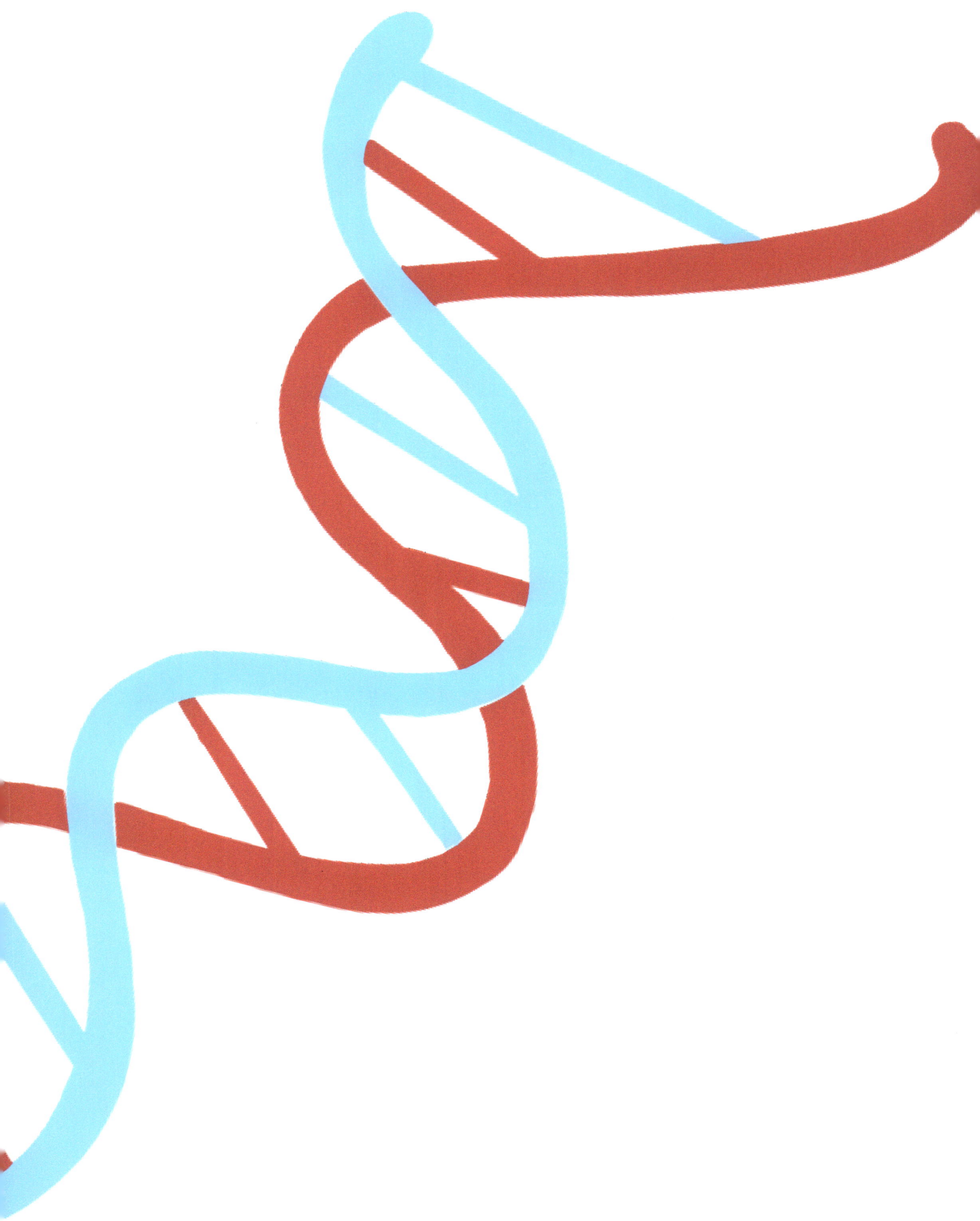

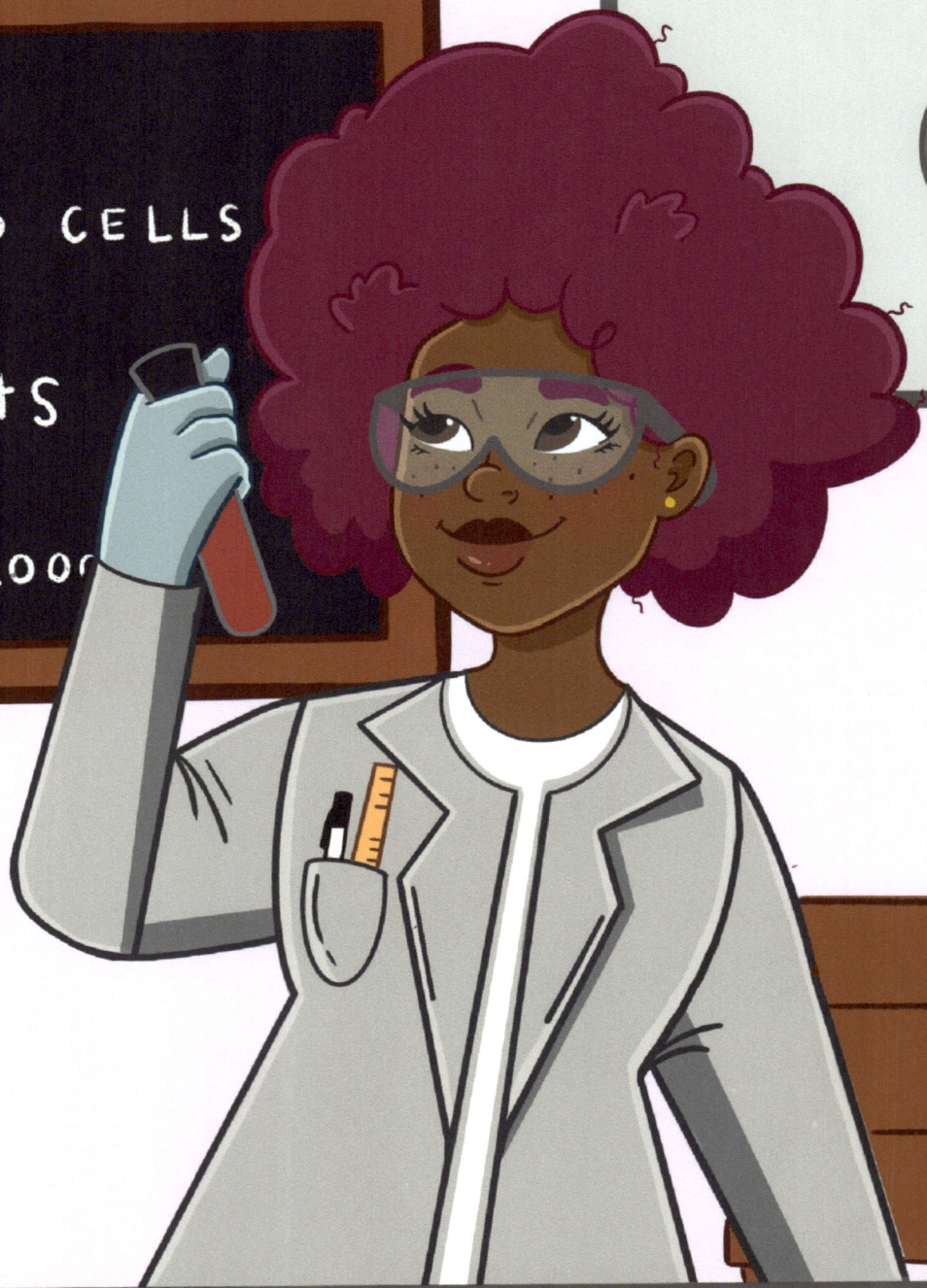

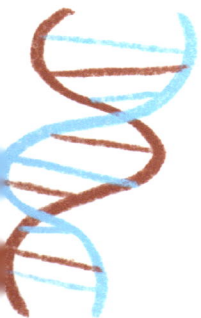

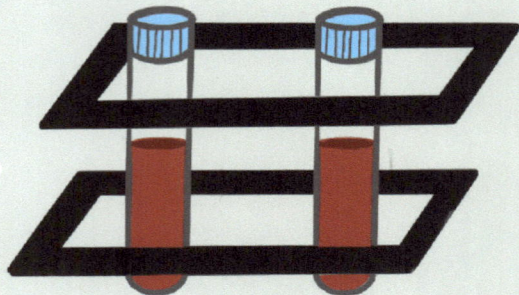

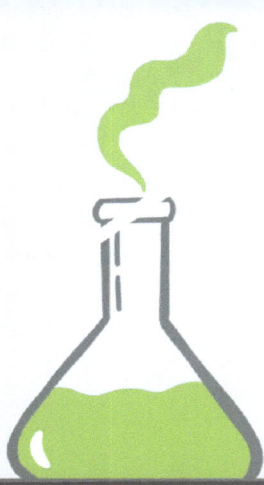

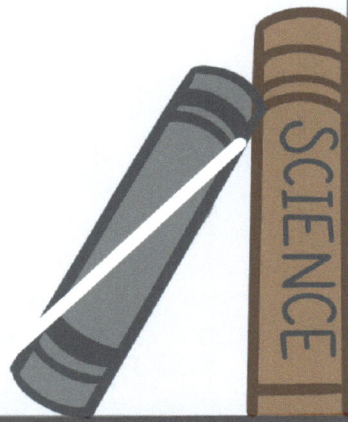

H is for Hematologist. A hematologist is a doctor that specializes in blood diseases, like Sickle Cell.

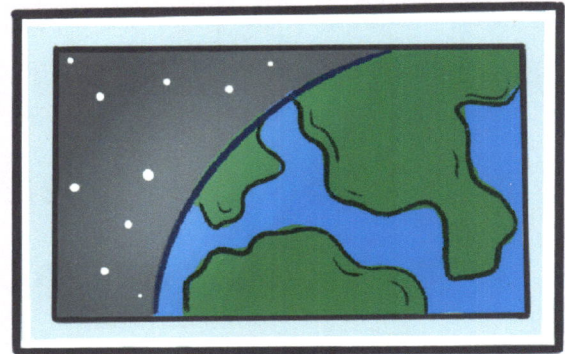

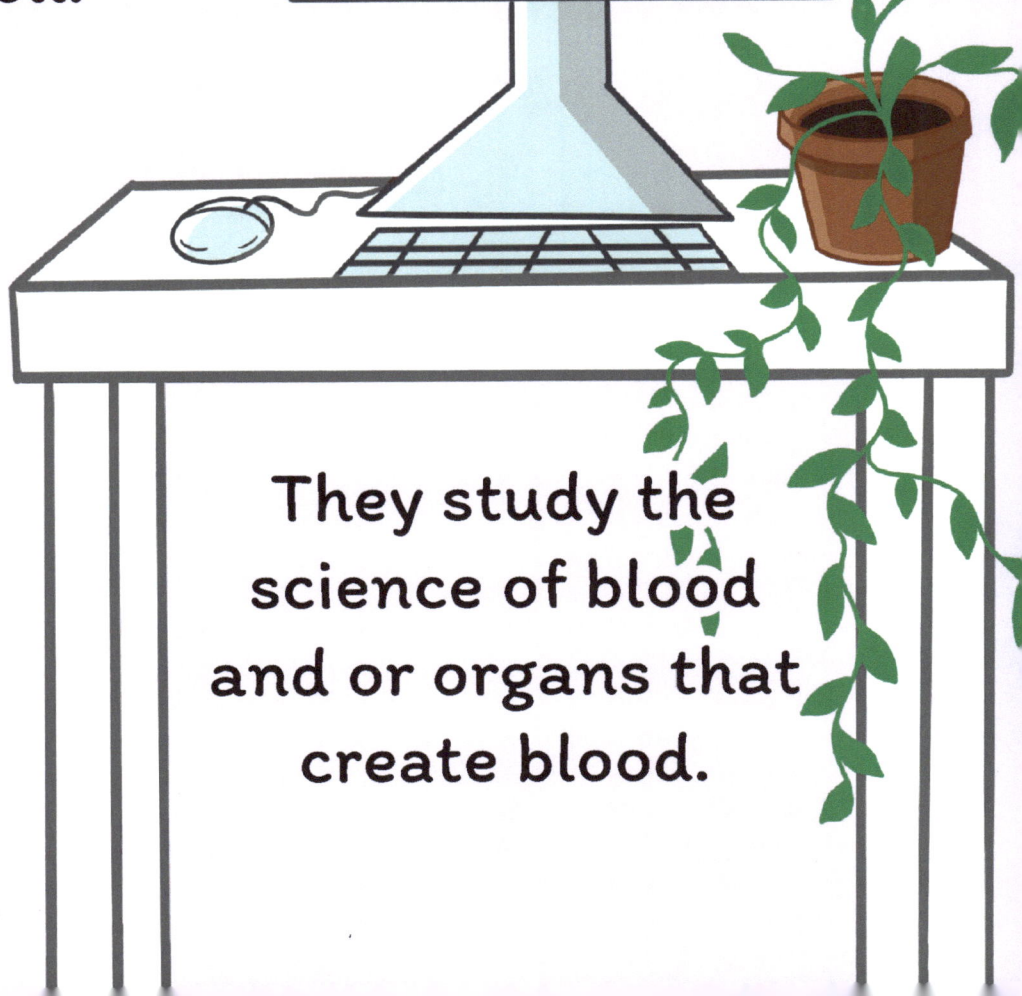

They study the science of blood and or organs that create blood.

I is for Infection.
With Sickle Cell there is an increased risk of developing infections like pneumonia, bloodstream infections, meningitis and bone infections. The immune system in Sickle Cell patients is not as strong as non-diseased patients.

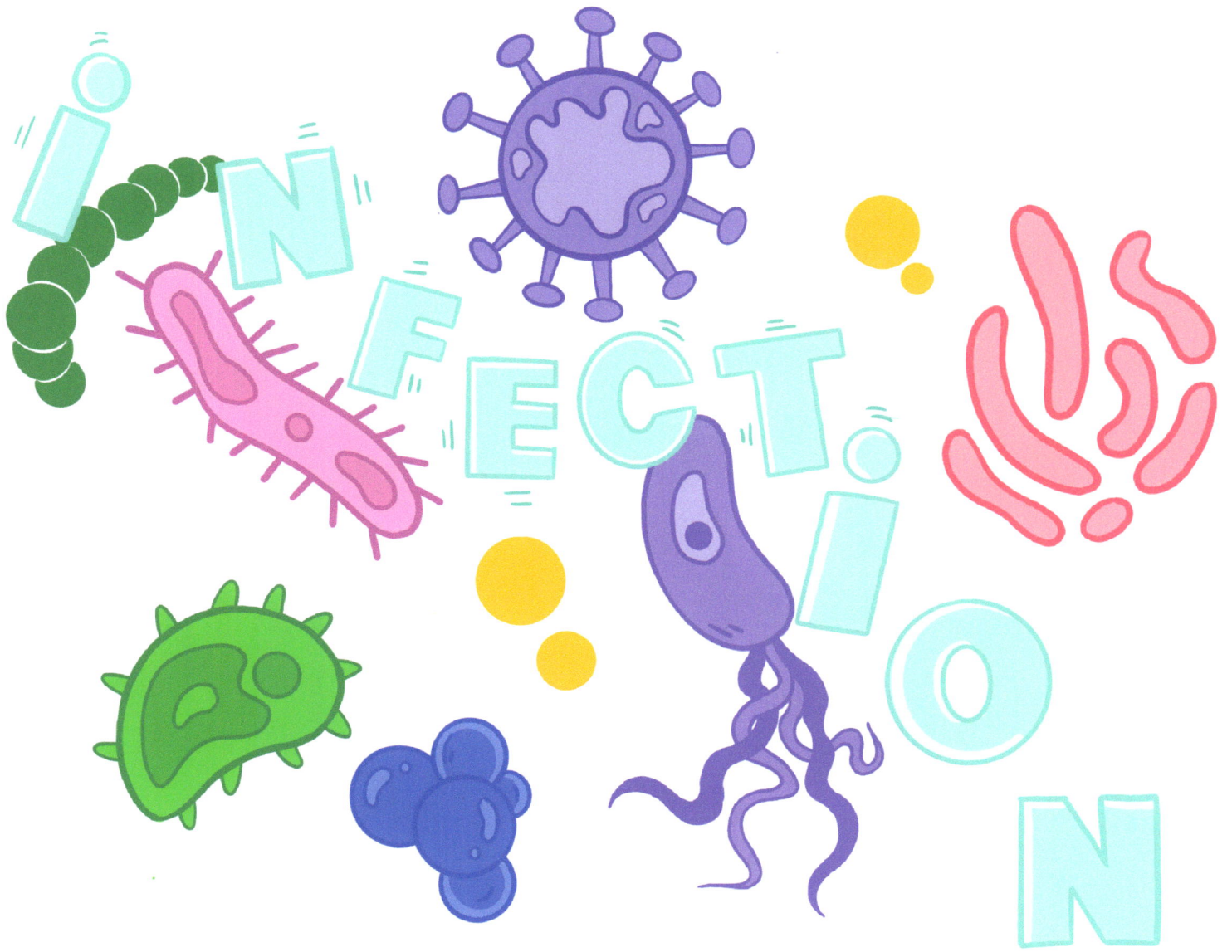

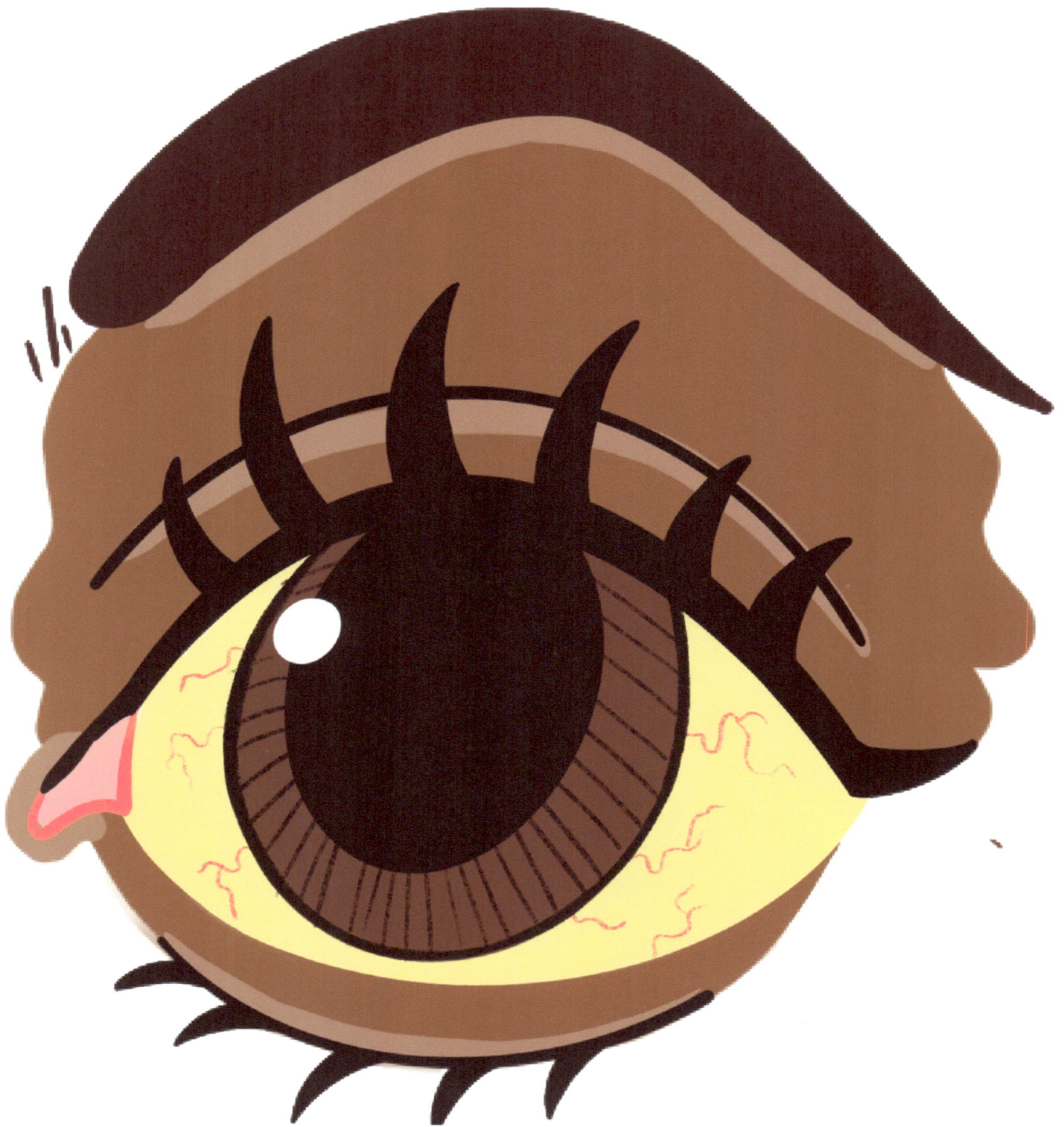

J is for Jaundice.
Sickle cells do not live as long as
normal red blood cells. They die at
a faster rate than the liver can filter
them out. Bilirubin from the broken
down cells gets built up in
the system, causing jaundice.

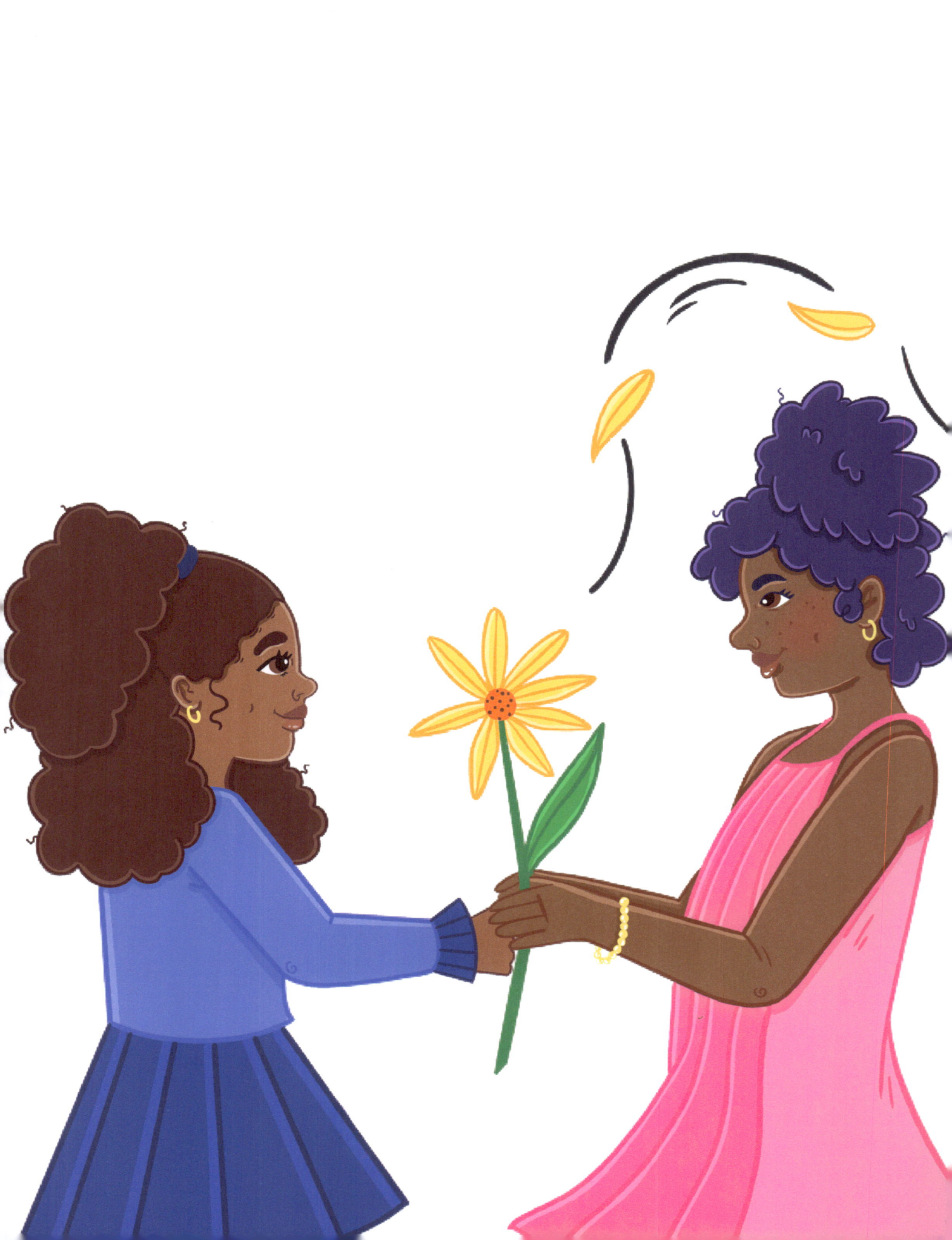

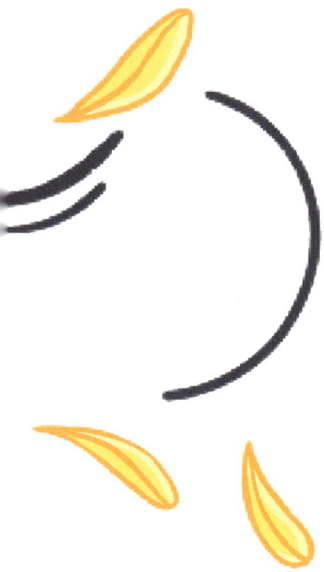

K is for Kindness.
Remember to always be kind.
We don't know what others are
going through.

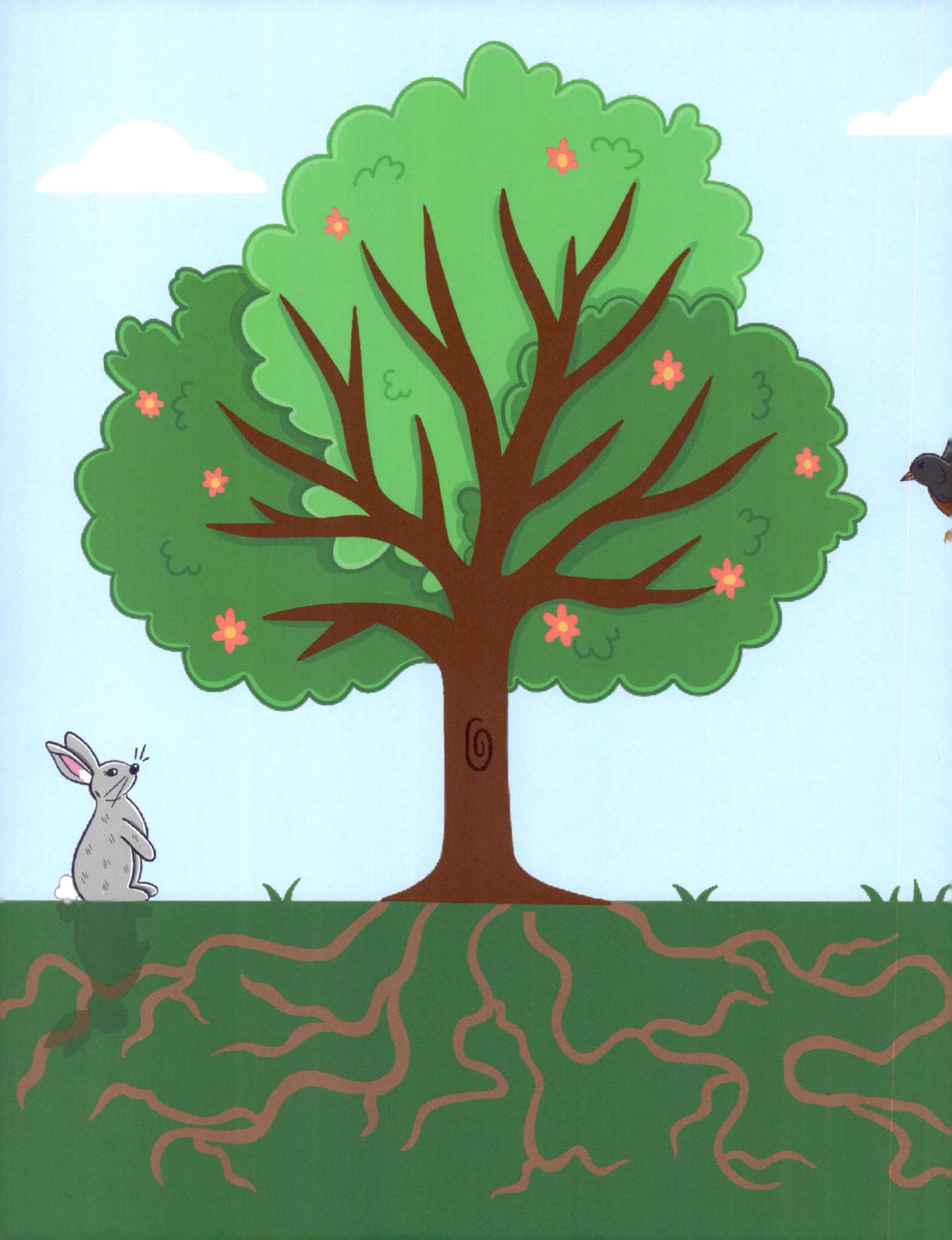

L is for Life. Life is precious, live it to the fullest.

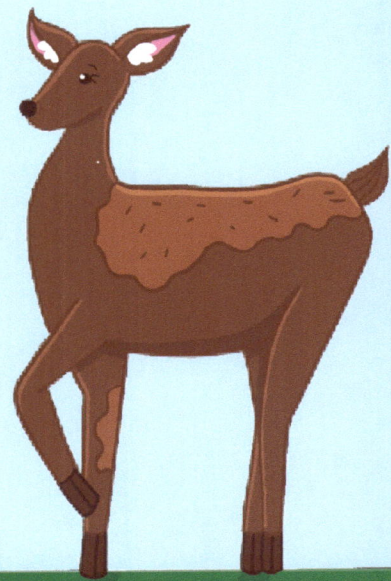

M is for Marrow.
A bone marrow transplant can actually cure Sickle Cell Disease.

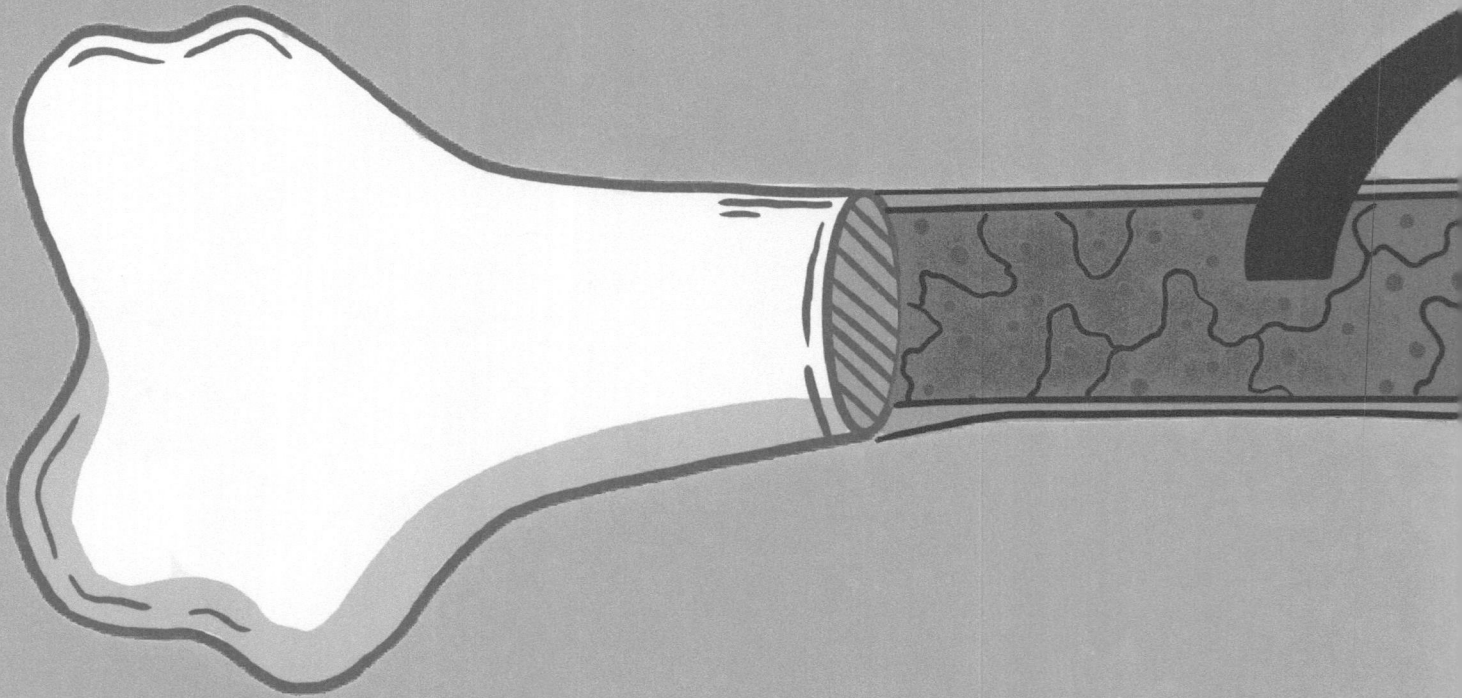

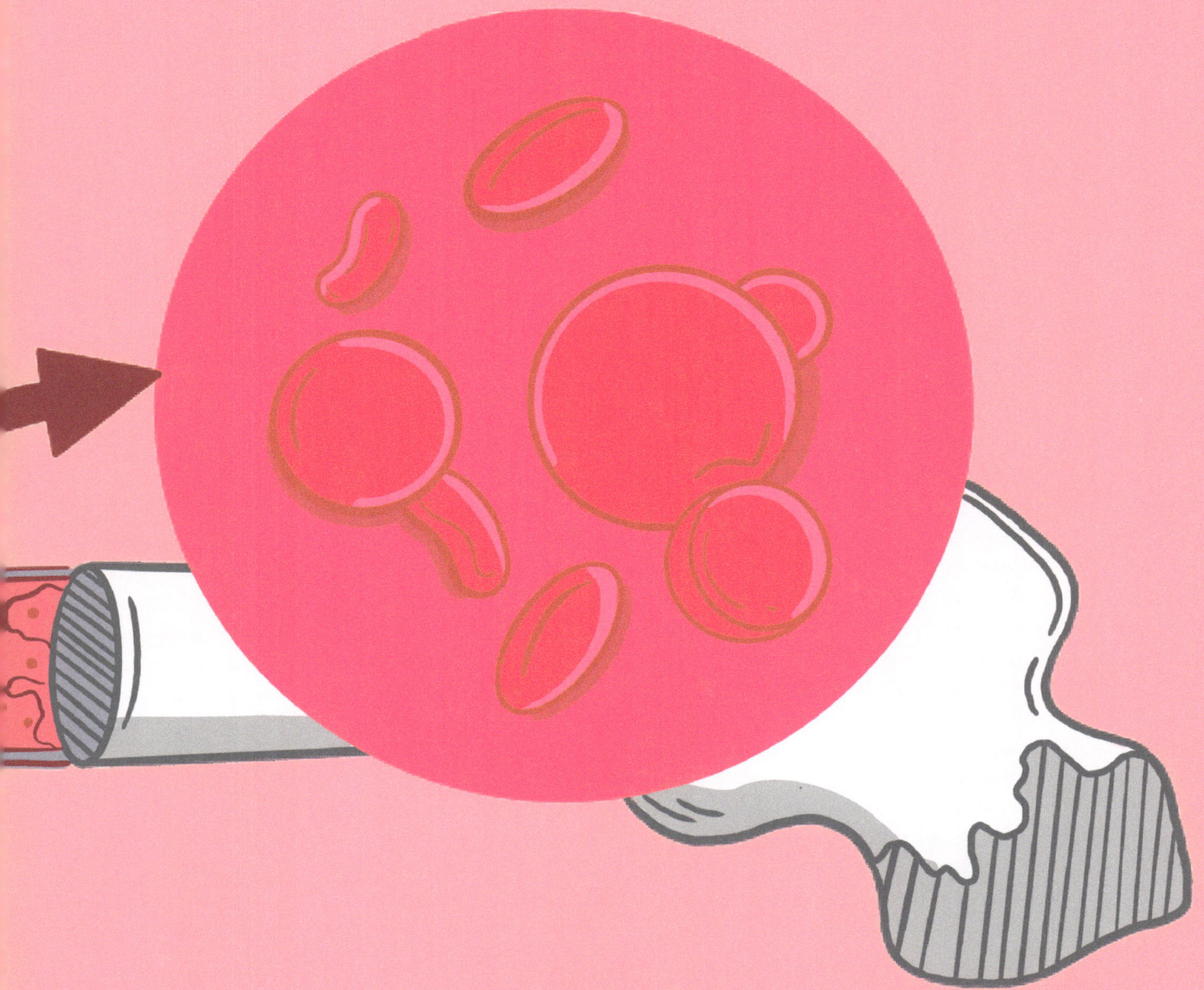

In this procedure,
healthy stem cells are used
to replace damaged ones.

N is for Newborn blood screening test. A blood test that looks for rare and serious health conditions (like Sickle Cell), usually conducted before the baby leaves the hospital.

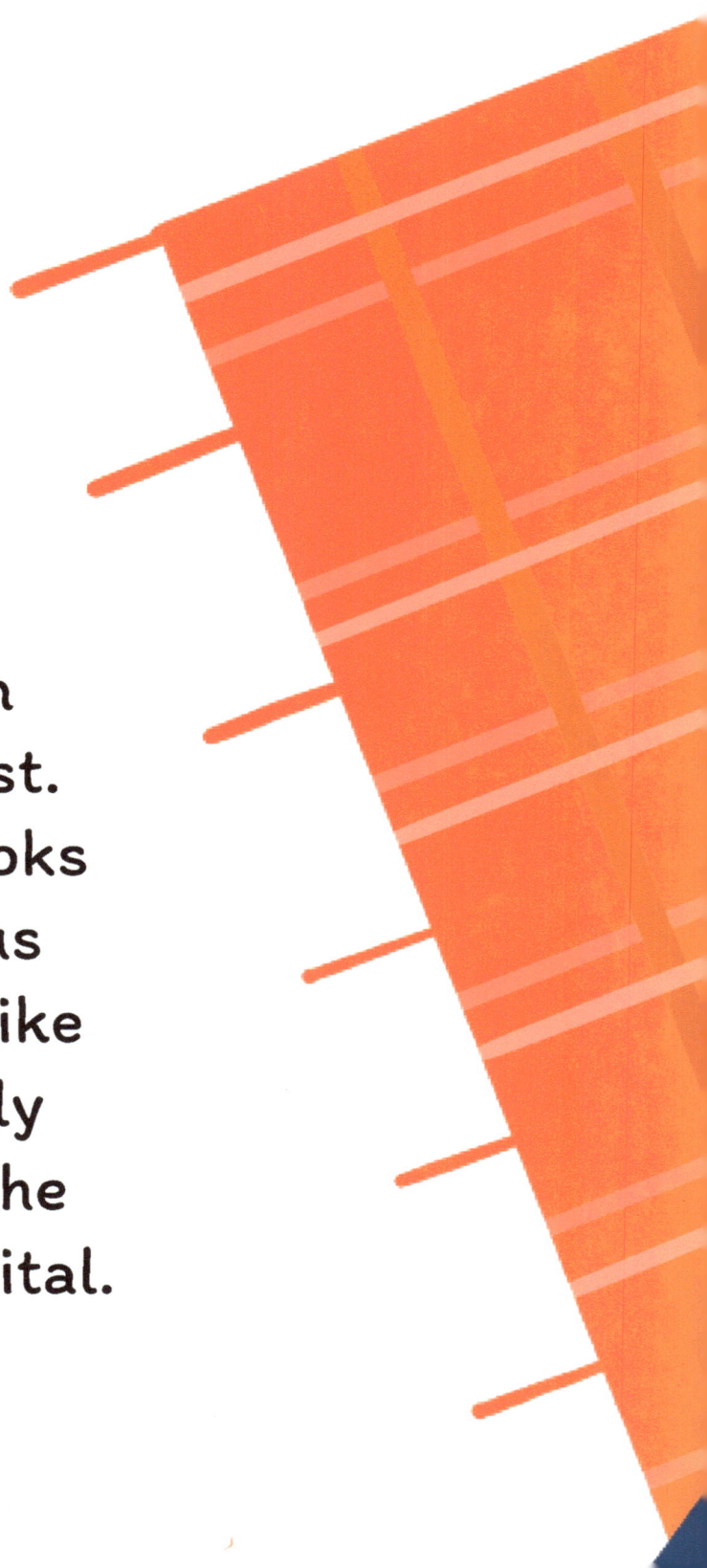

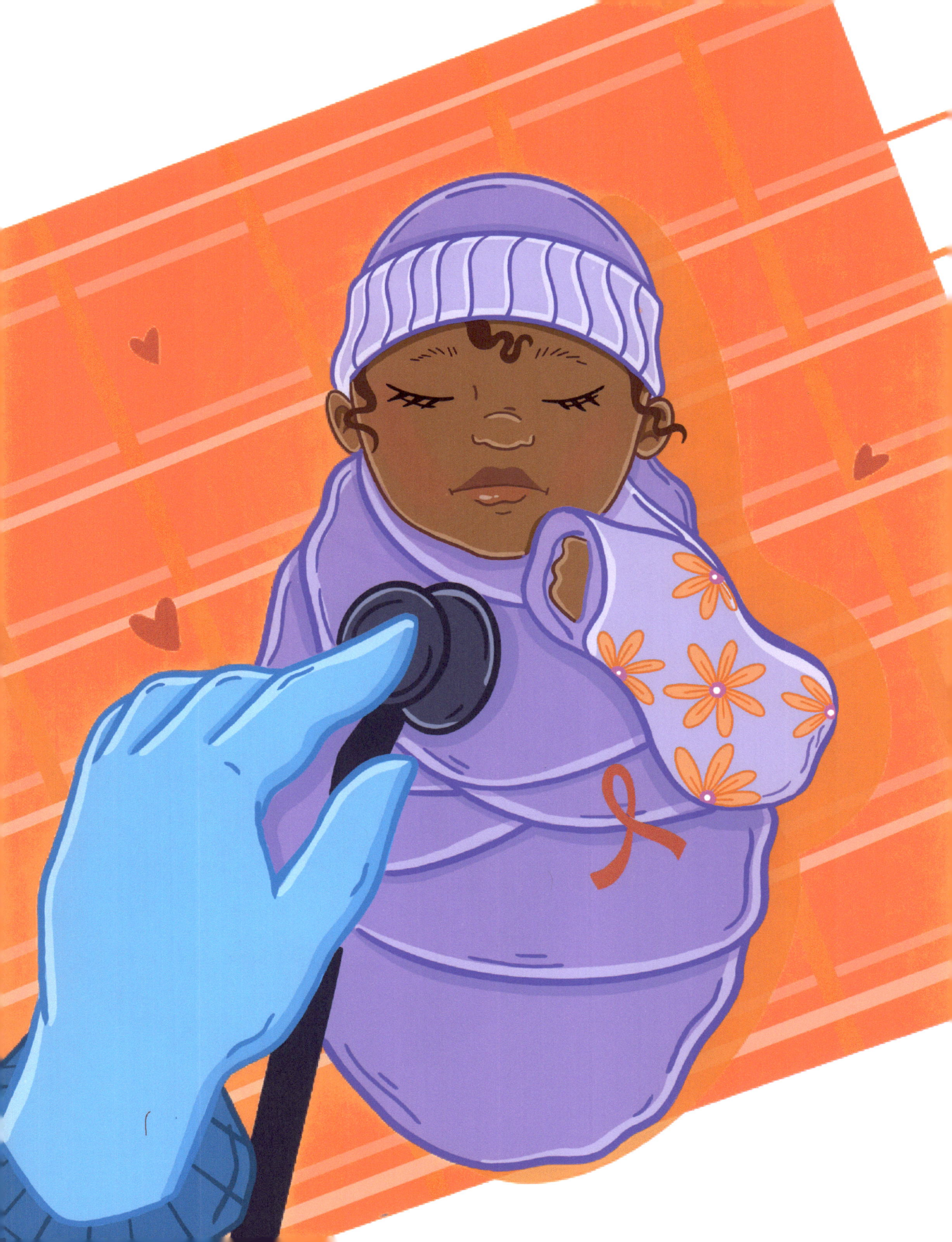

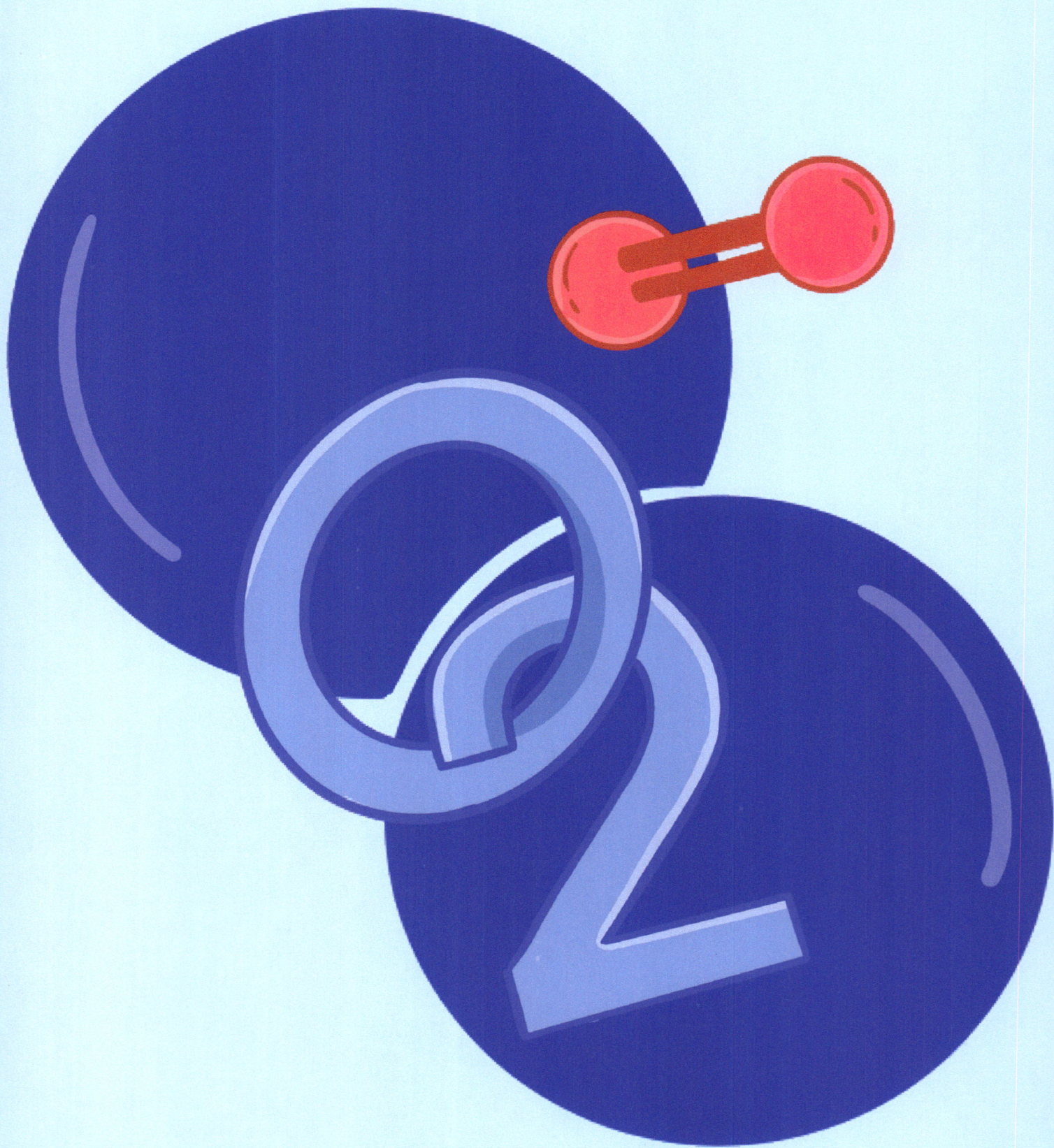

O is for Oxygen.
When normal red blood cells,
usually doughnut shaped,
lose oxygen they become banana,
C or sickle shaped. Hence the name
Sickle Cell Disease.

PAIN
CRISI

P is for Pain crisis.
Pain crisis aka Sickle Cell crisis
happens when pain comes suddenly
and can persist for hours, as a result
of sickle red blood cells blocking
blood flow to bones.

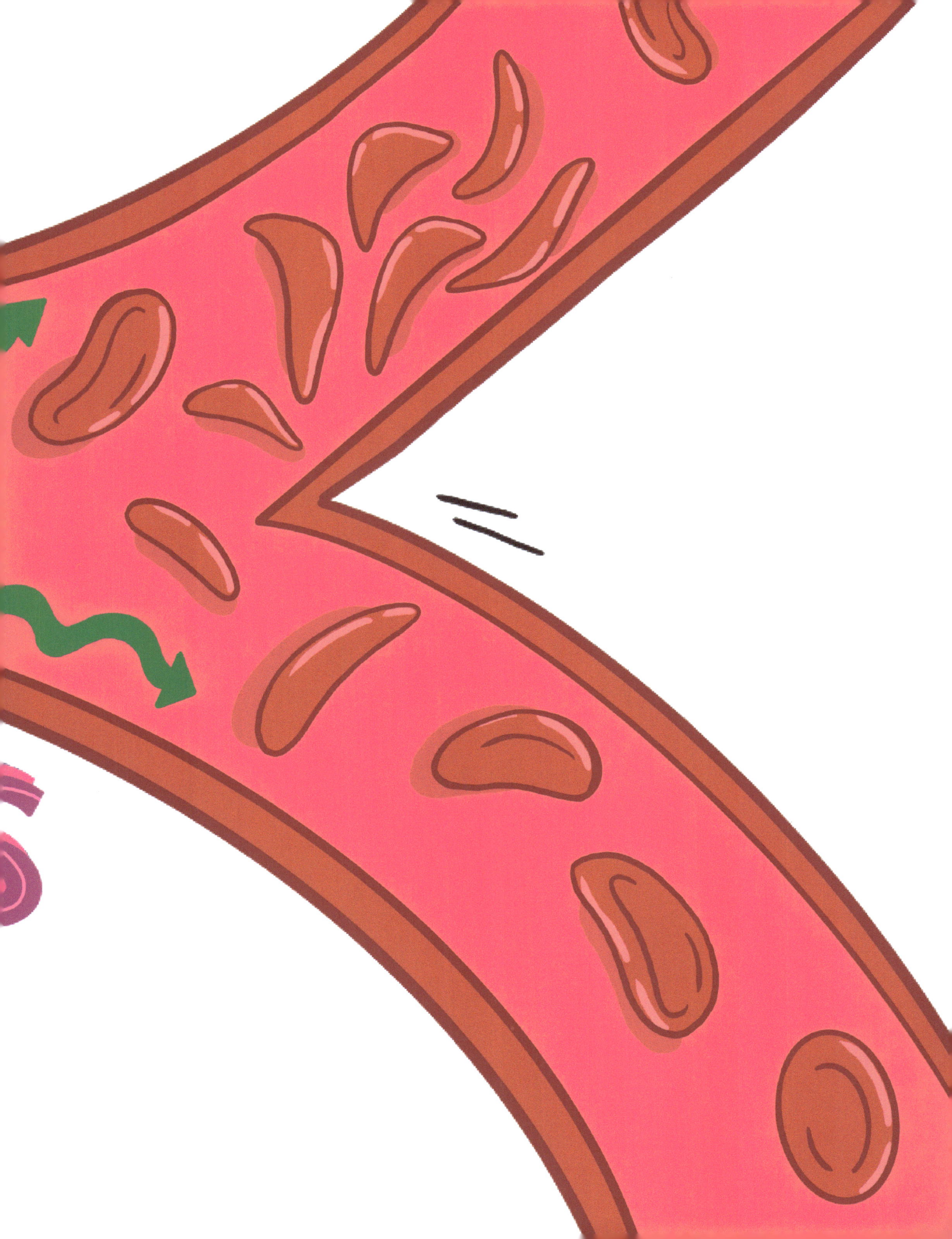

Q is for Quick.
Quick response to any
symptoms of Sickle Cell
complications or crisis is so
important in finding and
treating the issue.

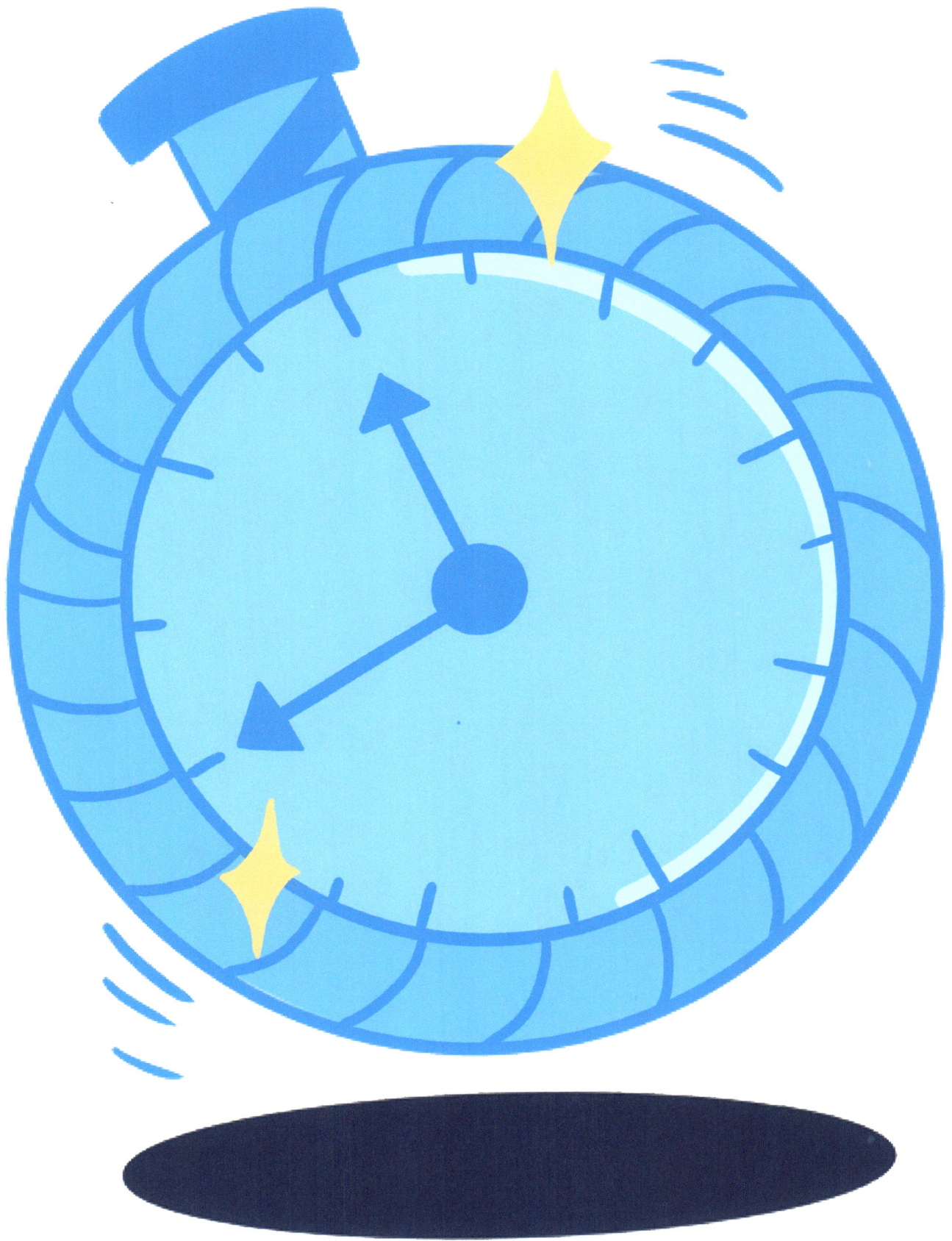

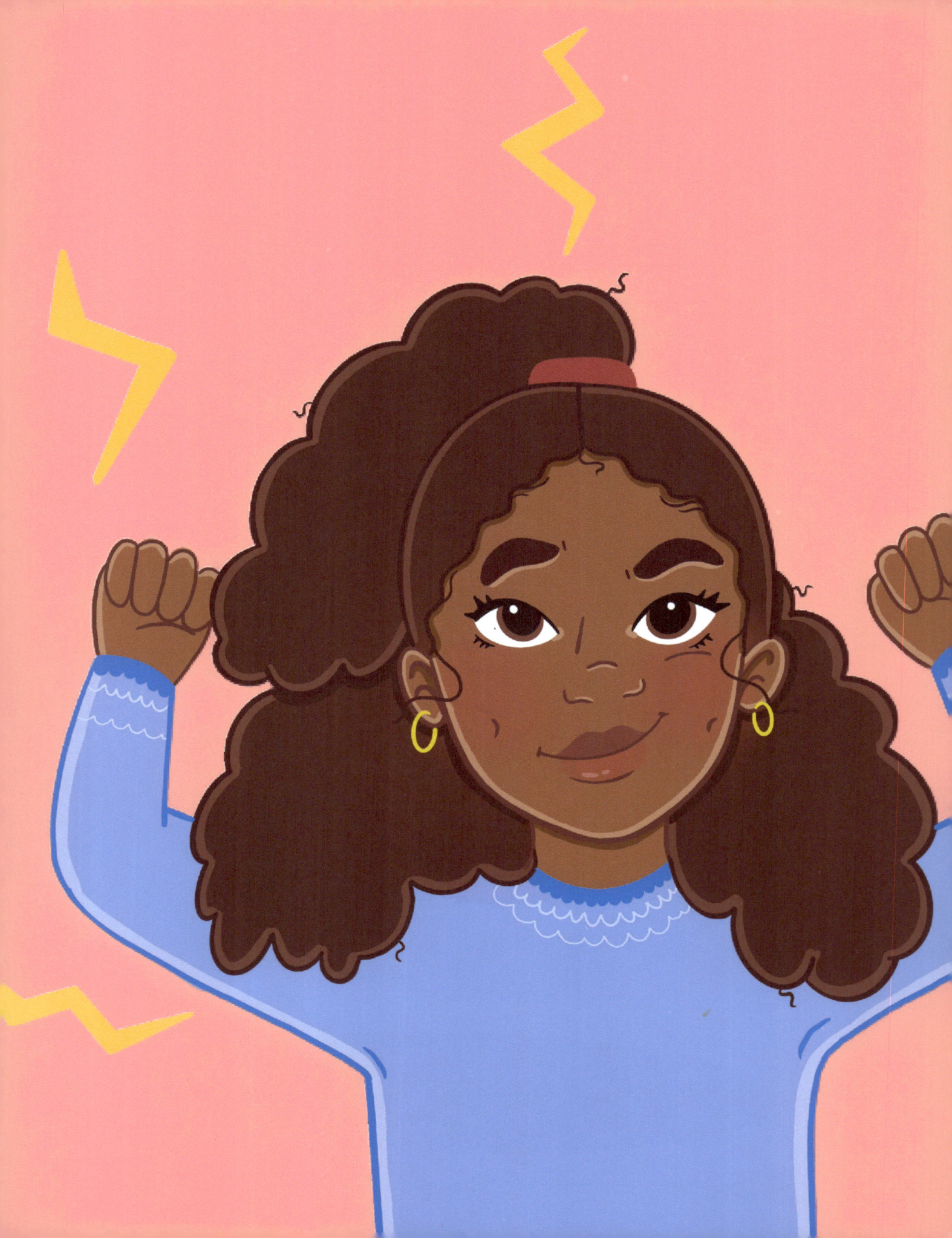

R is for Resilient.
Anyone with Sickle Cell
Disease is resilient. We are able
to withstand and recover
from difficulties.

S is for Spleen.
With Sickle Cell the spleen
does not operate correctly.
The spleen filters bacteria from the
bloodstream and produces antibodies.
The sickle cells clog the blood vessels
in the spleen, which lead to damage
and poor protection against infection.
It's common for Sickle Cell patients
to have their spleen taken out.

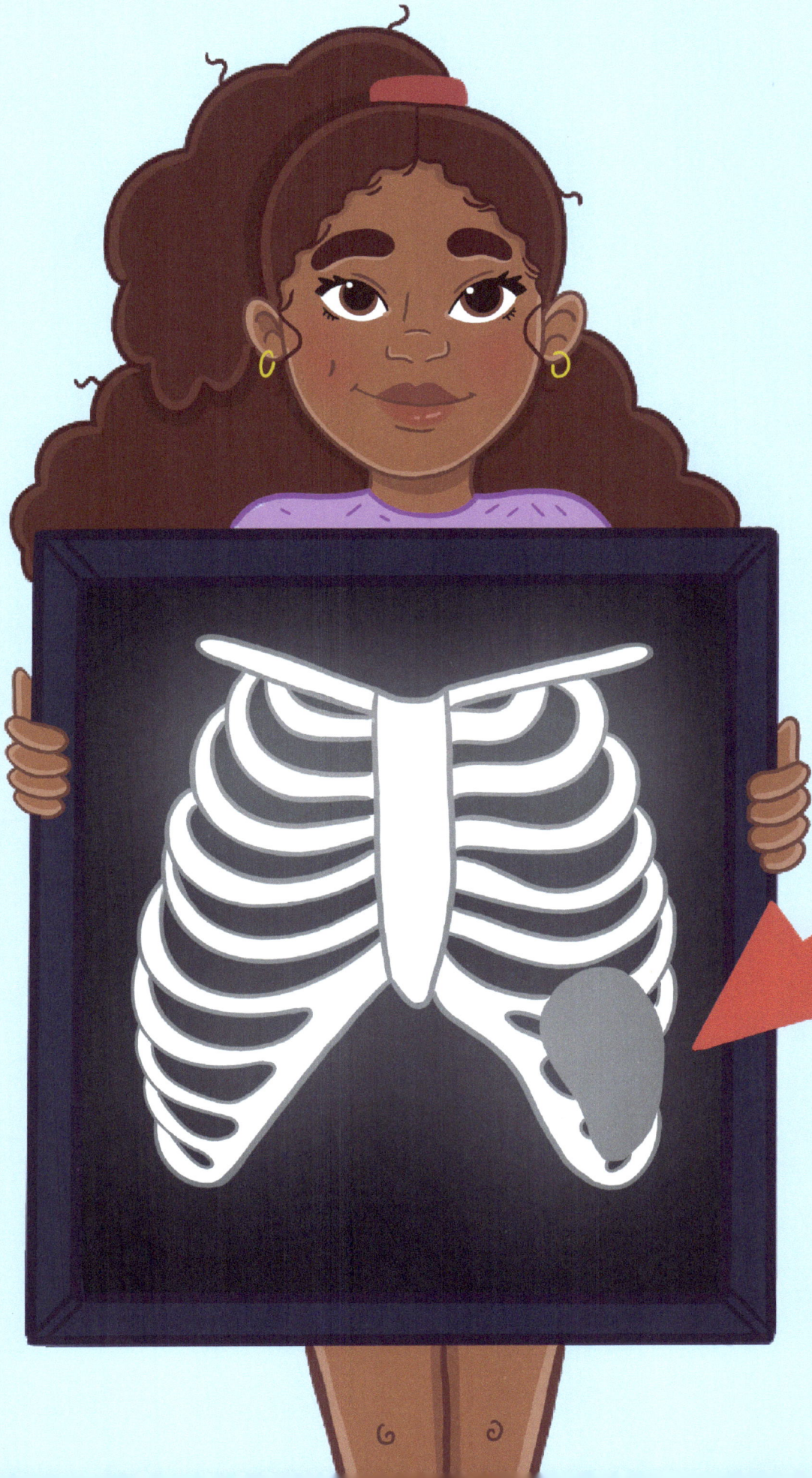

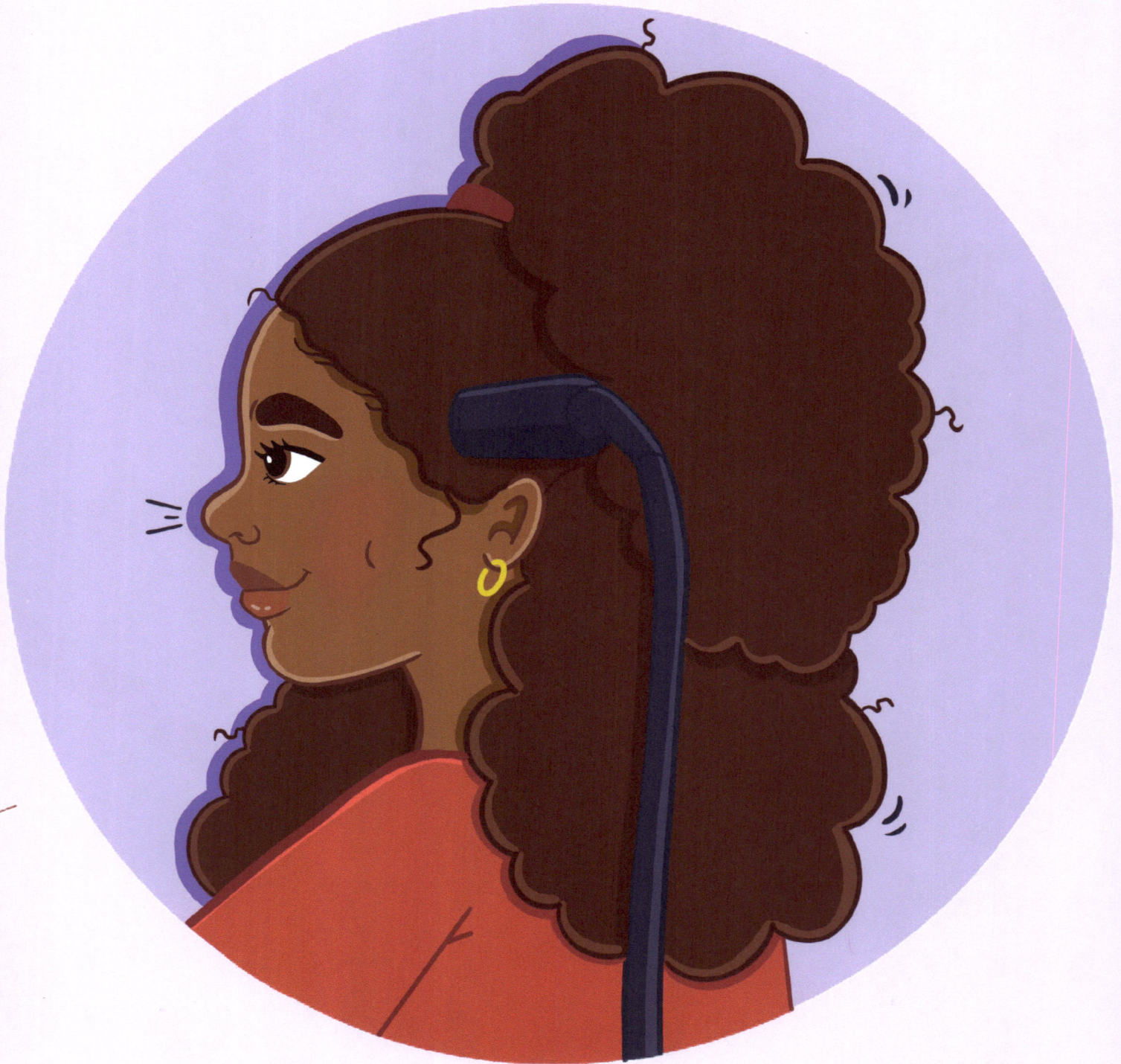

T is for Transcranial Doppler or TCD.
A TCD is an ultrasound that
screens for strokes in children
with Sickle Cell Disease.

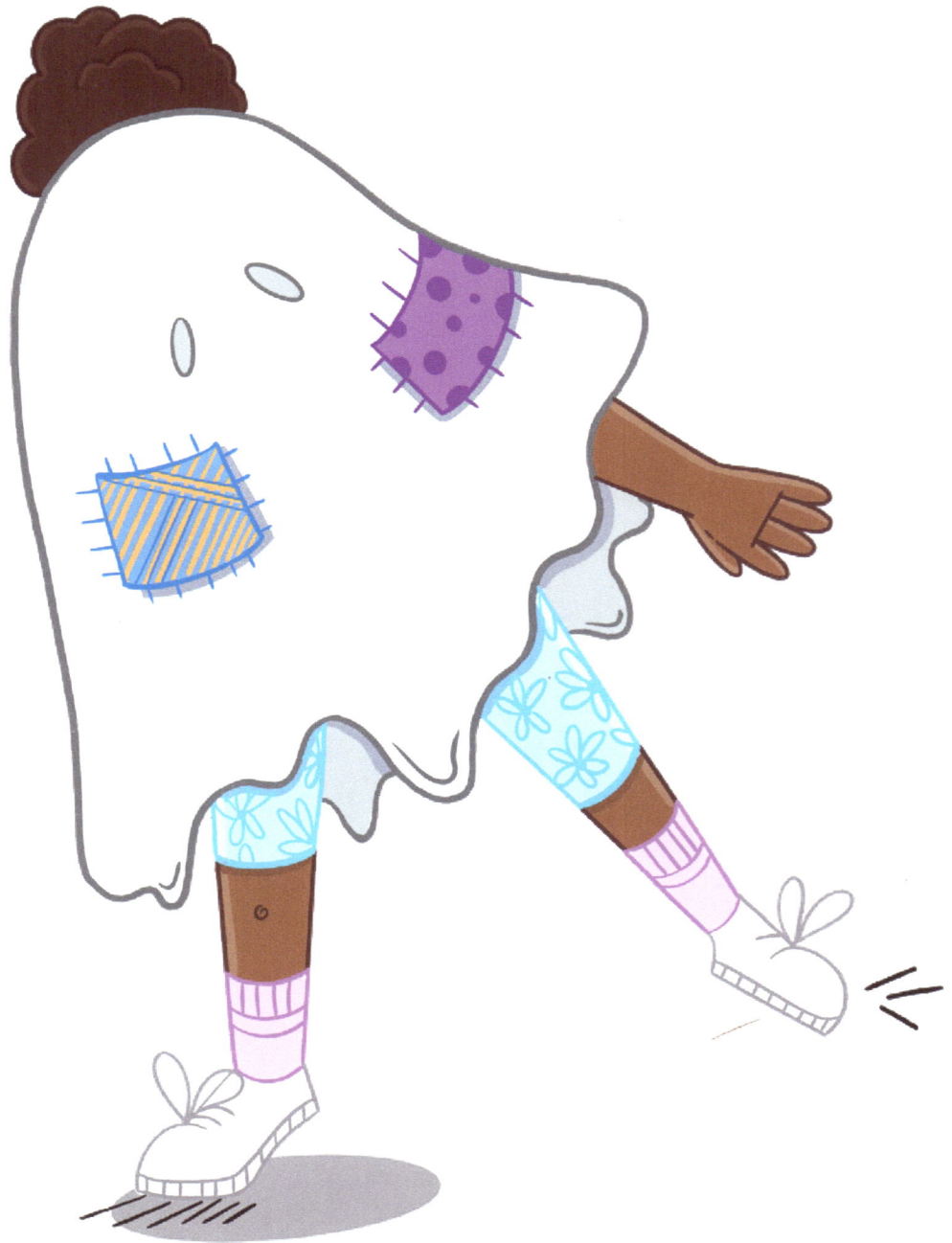

U is for Unseen.
Most Sickle Cell complications are unable to be seen, it takes tests to pin point exactly what's going on.

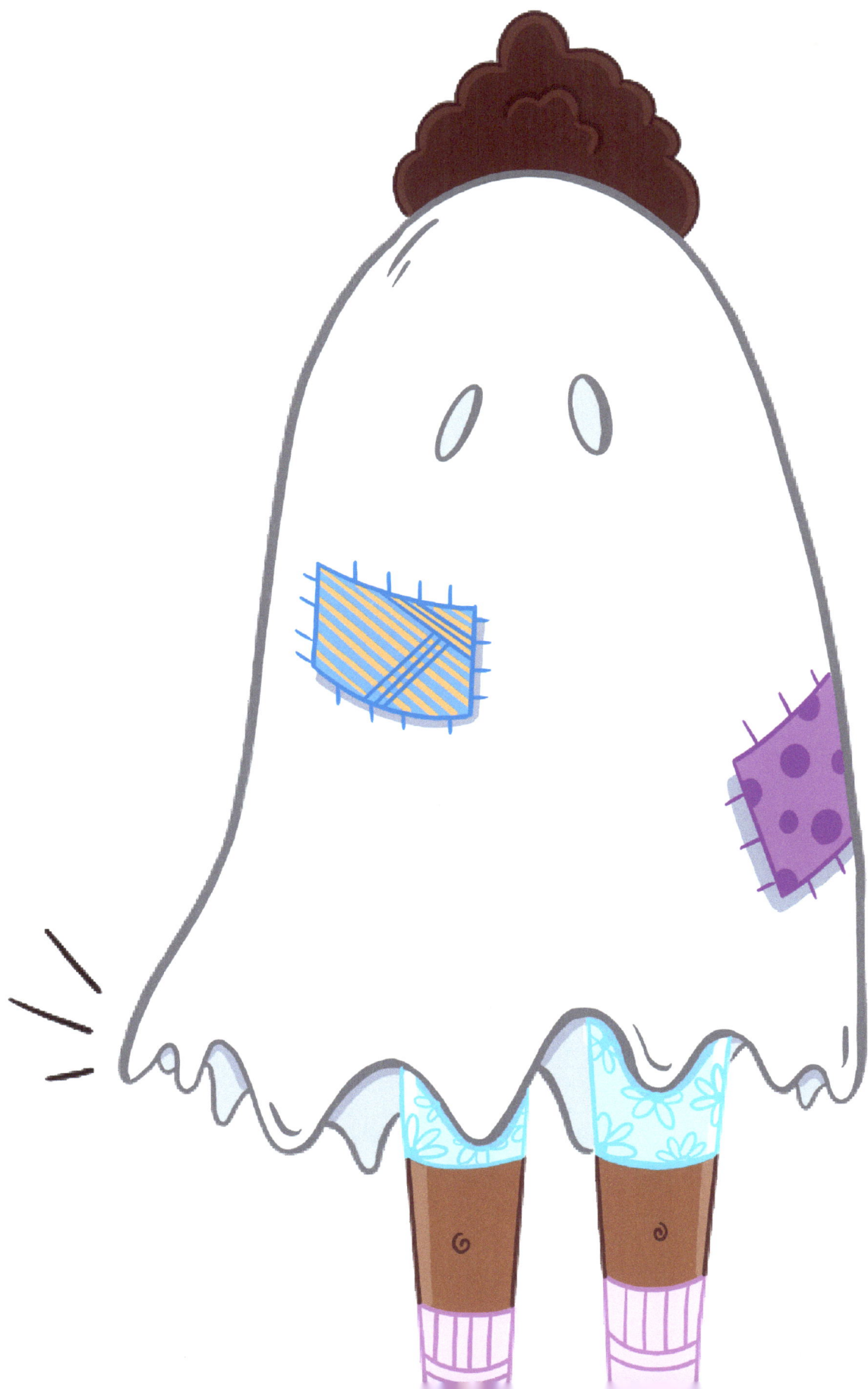

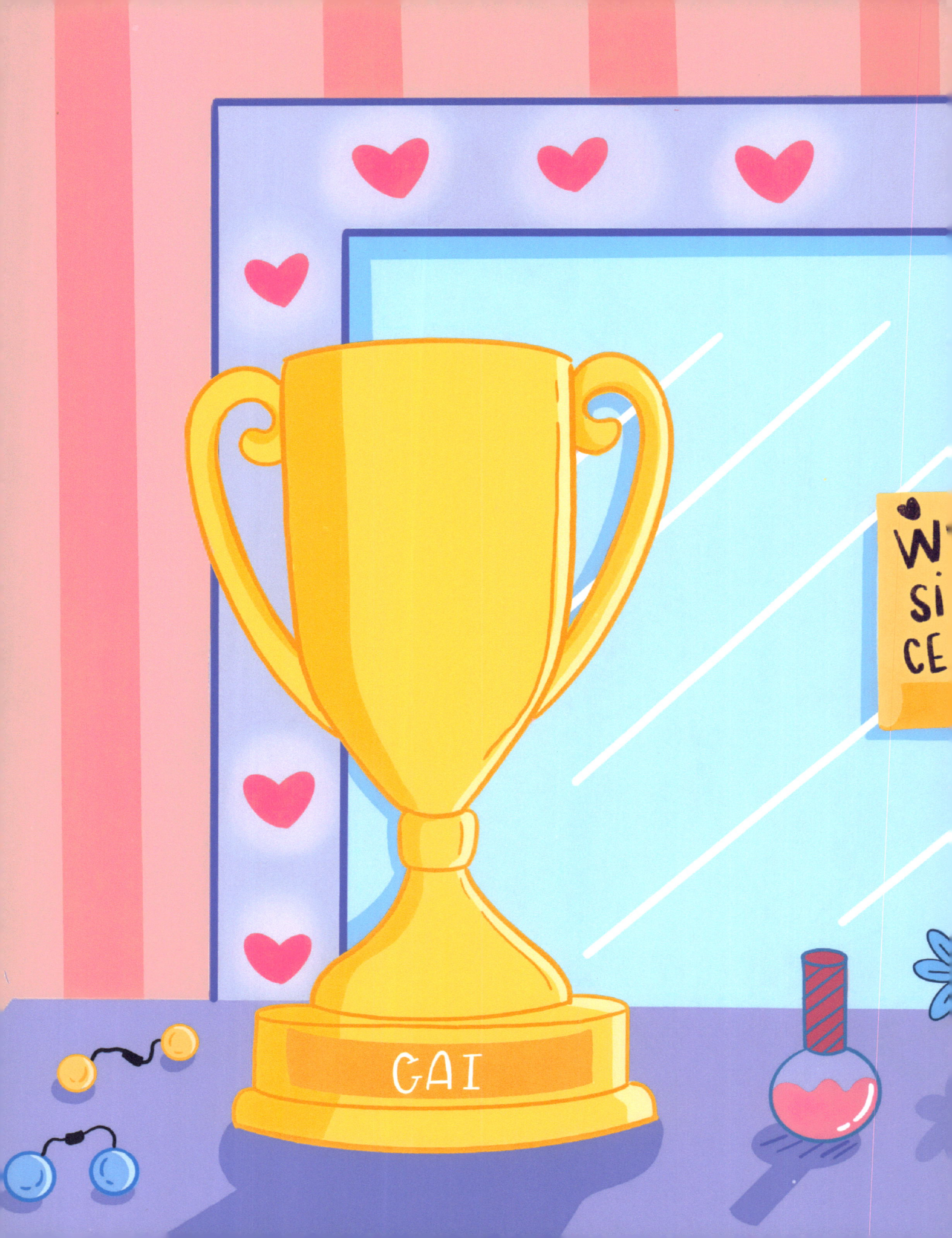

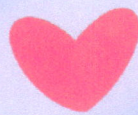

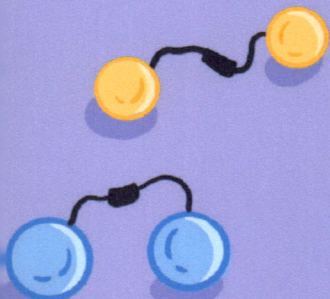

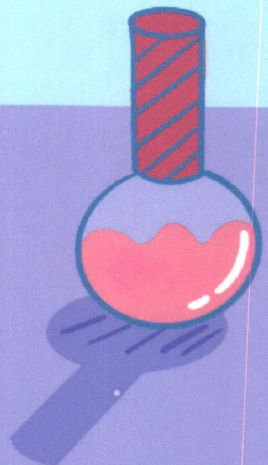

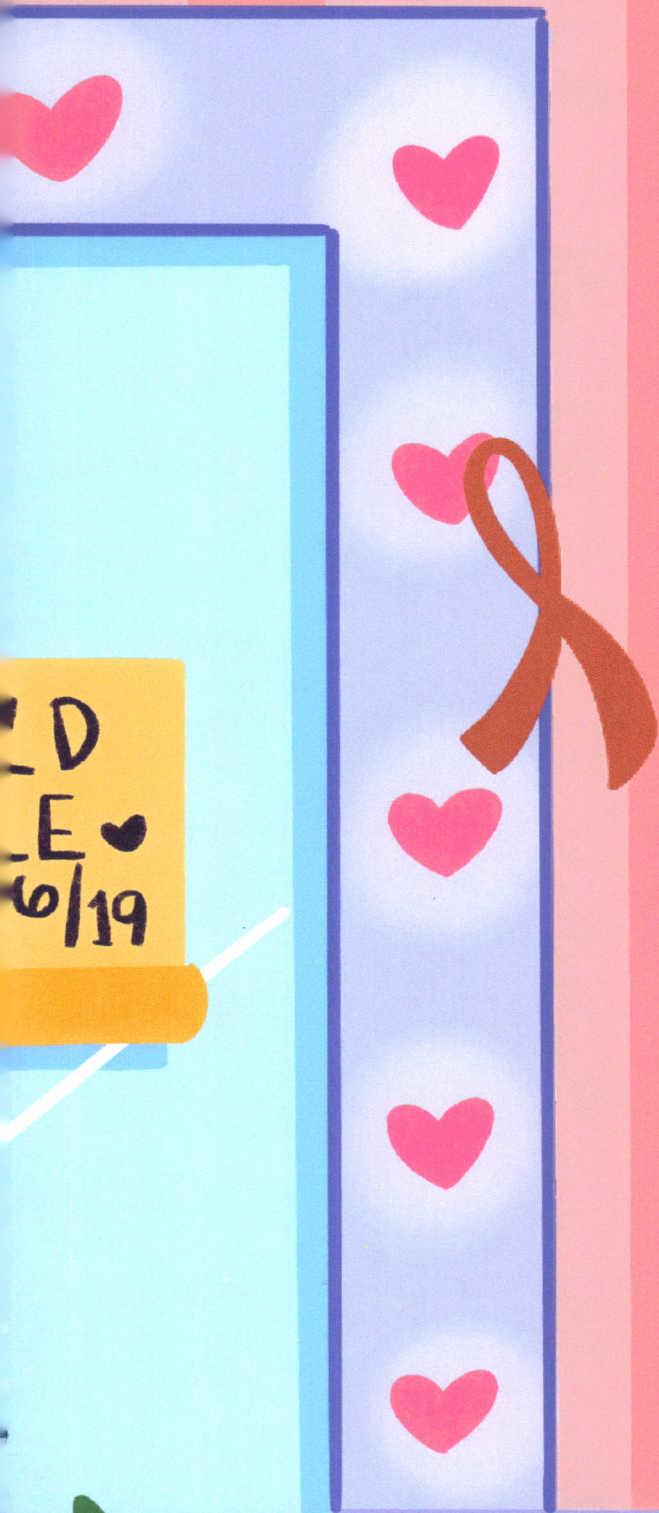

V is for Victorious.
We, Sickle Cell warriors,
are victorious in our
fight everyday!

W is for World.
World Sickle Cell day
is June 19th.

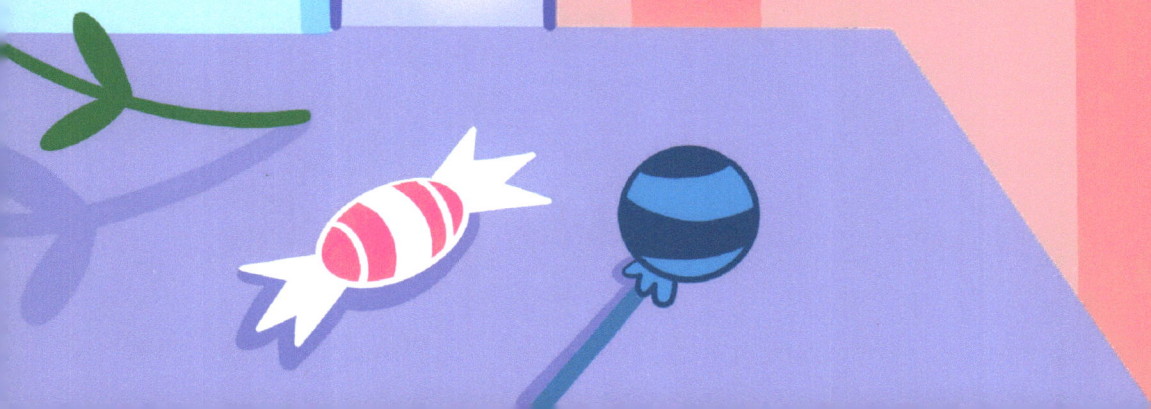

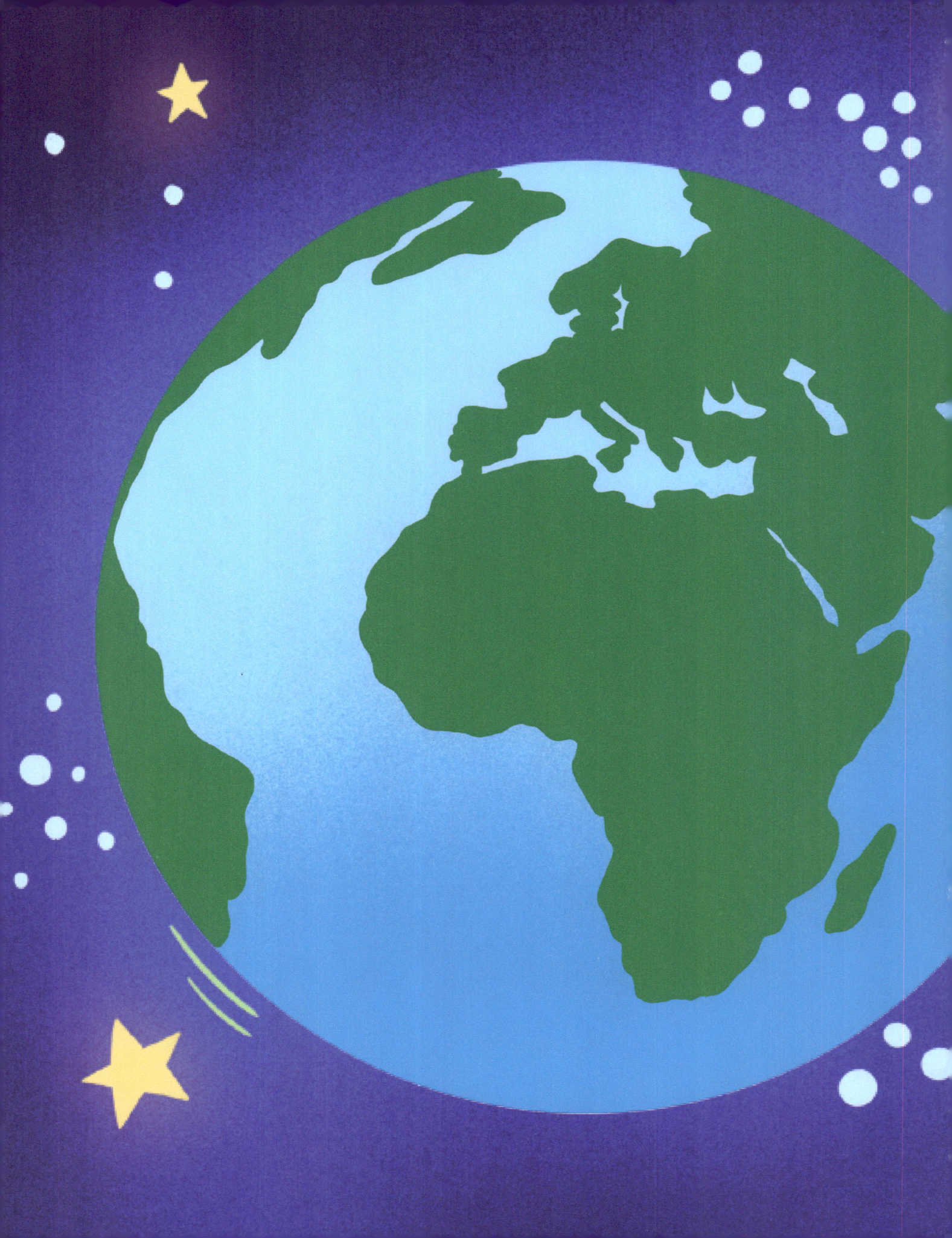

X is for eXist.
Exist like there
are no limitations.
Sickle Cell is not
our limit.

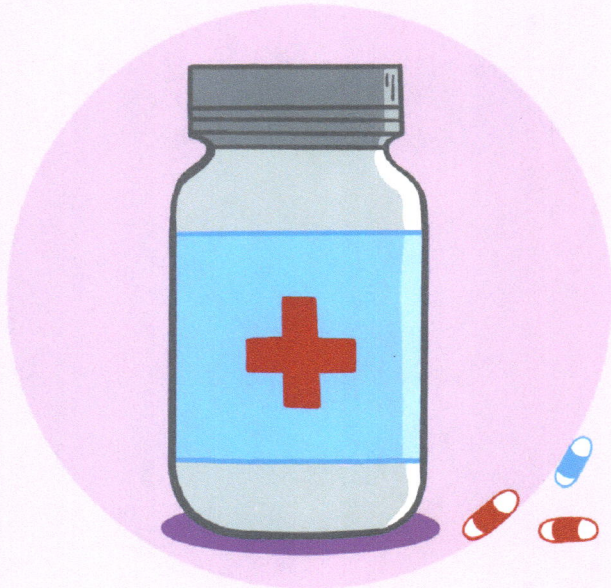

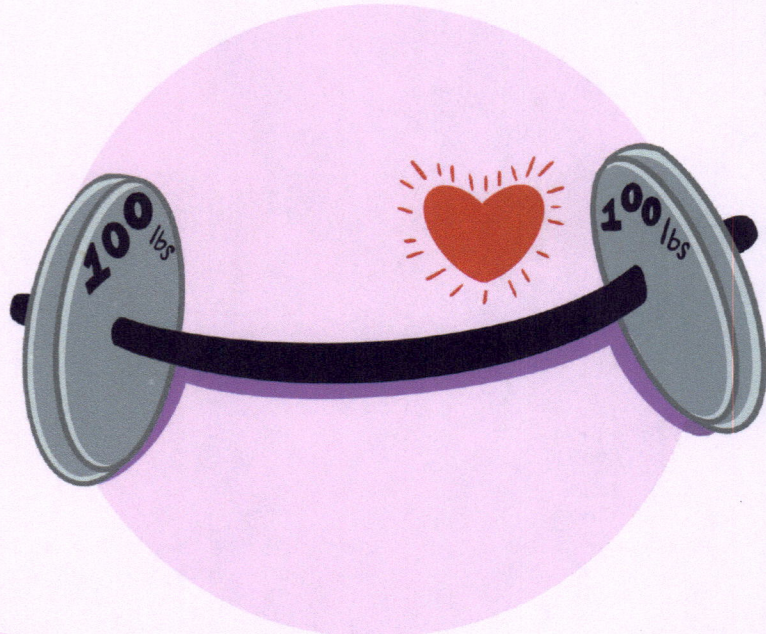

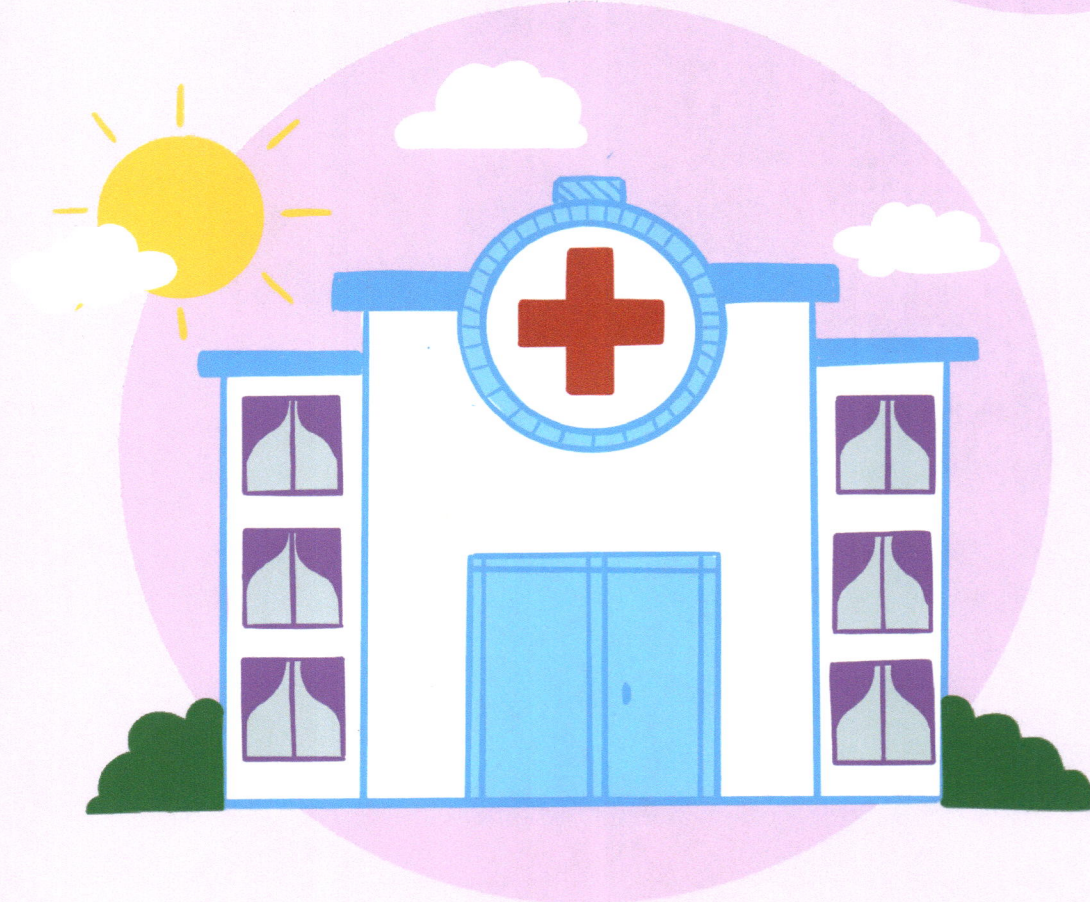

Y is for Youth.
Creating healthy habits and routines in Sickle Cell youth help us lead a great adult life.

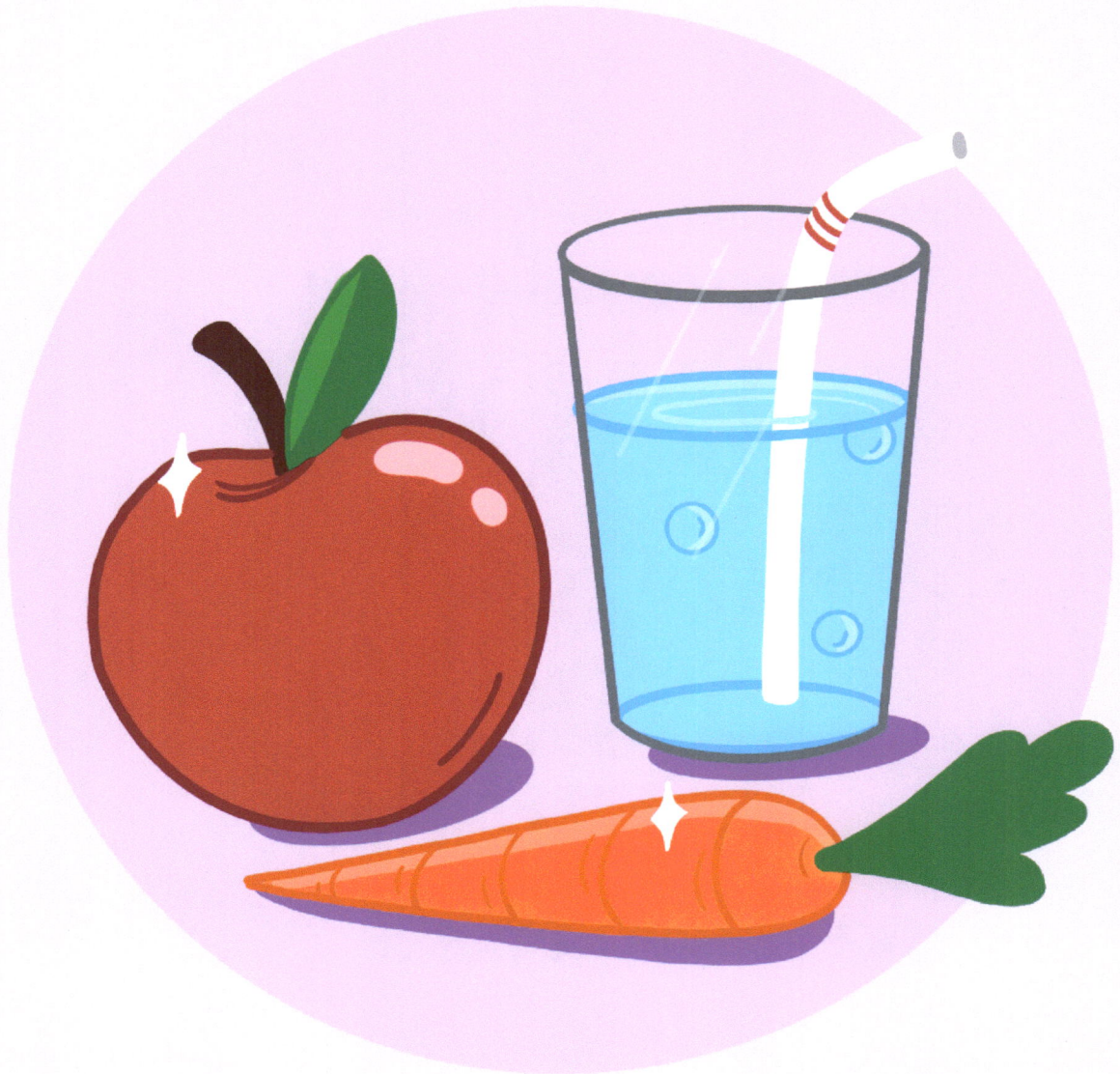

Z is for Zeal.

I, Cai have a zeal for life and teaching others about Sickle Cell Disease.

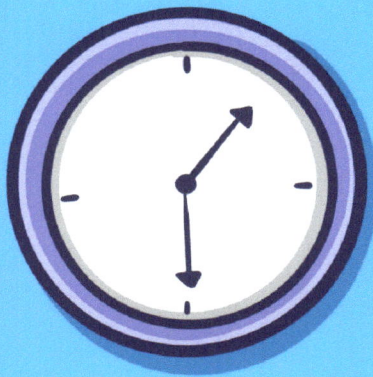

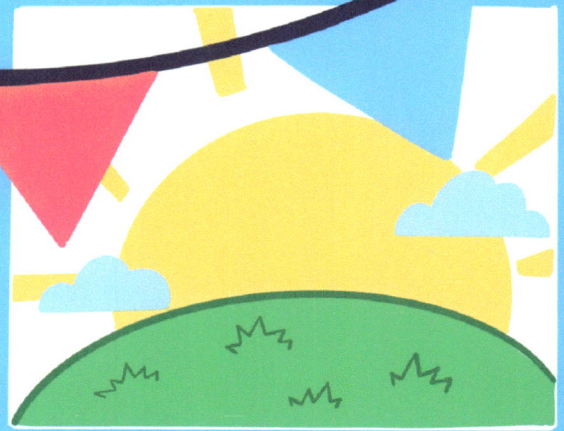

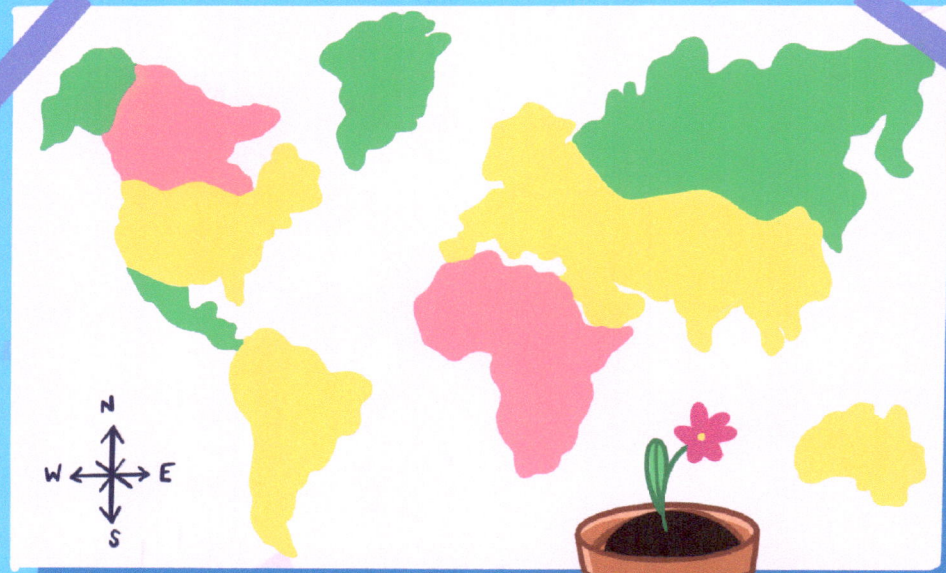

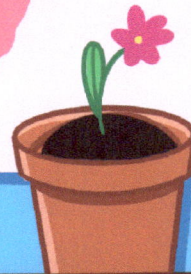

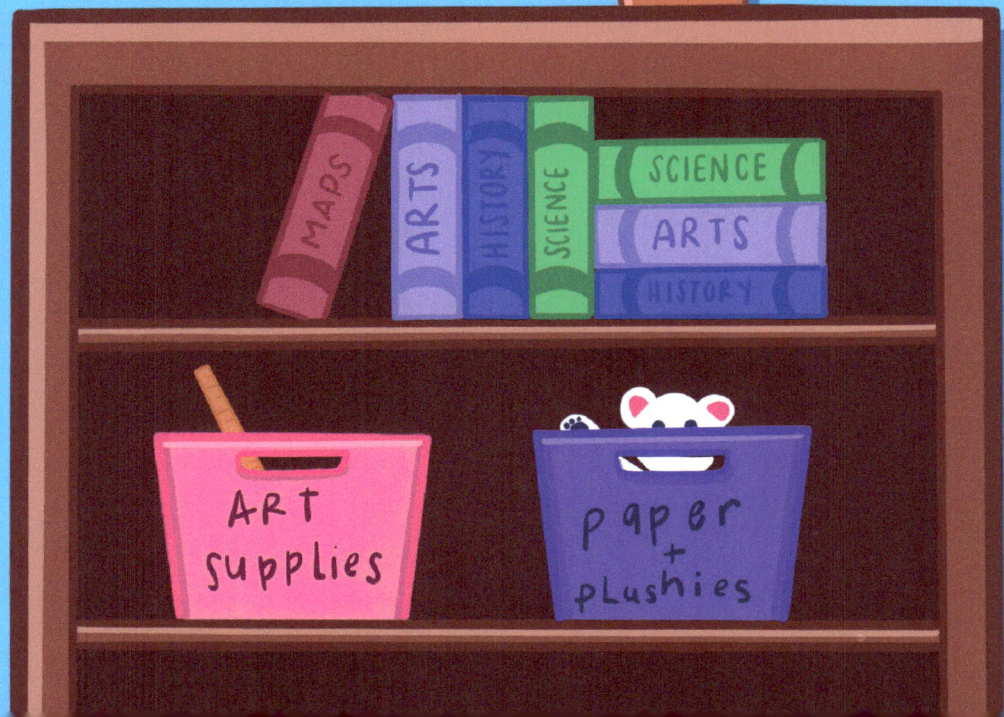

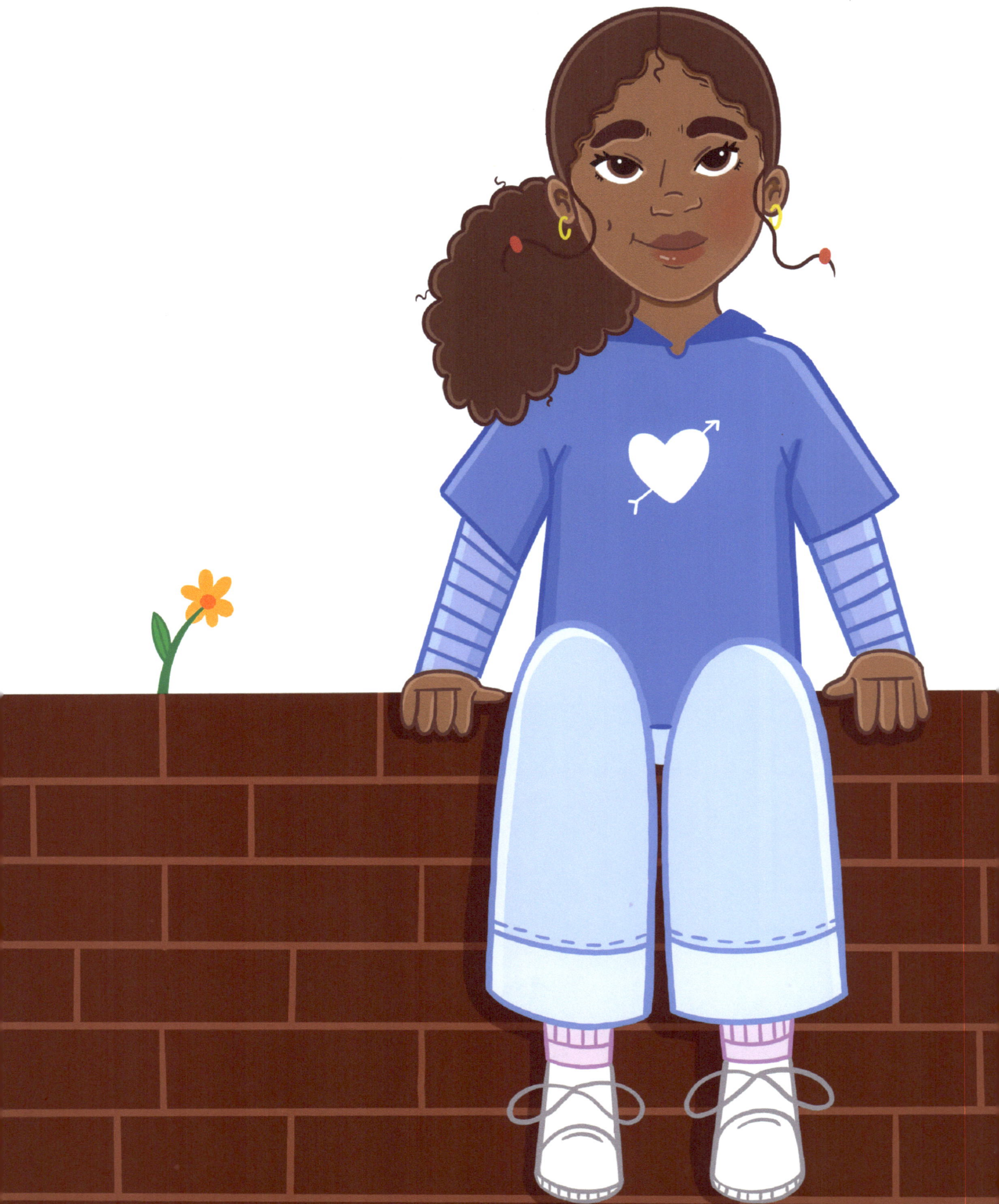

My amazing CaiBean! The previous statement is not just because she's my granddaughter it is because she truly is amazing. Amazing is what she was when she was born with a broken collarbone, then to find out she was born Sickle Cell. A rare form I might add. I have watched her grow, her personality develop with tenacity, energy like that of the energizer bunny, charisma, fearlessness, and a very loud voice! LOL which I believe was ordained to her DNA by God to deal with all of the hospital visits and stays, all of the pokes as she will call them from getting her blood drawn, all of the medication and changes in their dosages, the times of dealing with pain, weakness and not to mention high fevers. Through it all she still finds a way to be full of sunshine and rainbows, strength and resilience! This is why she is my amazing CaiBean. This is why She is CaiStrong.
I love your face forever
-Love you to life TT

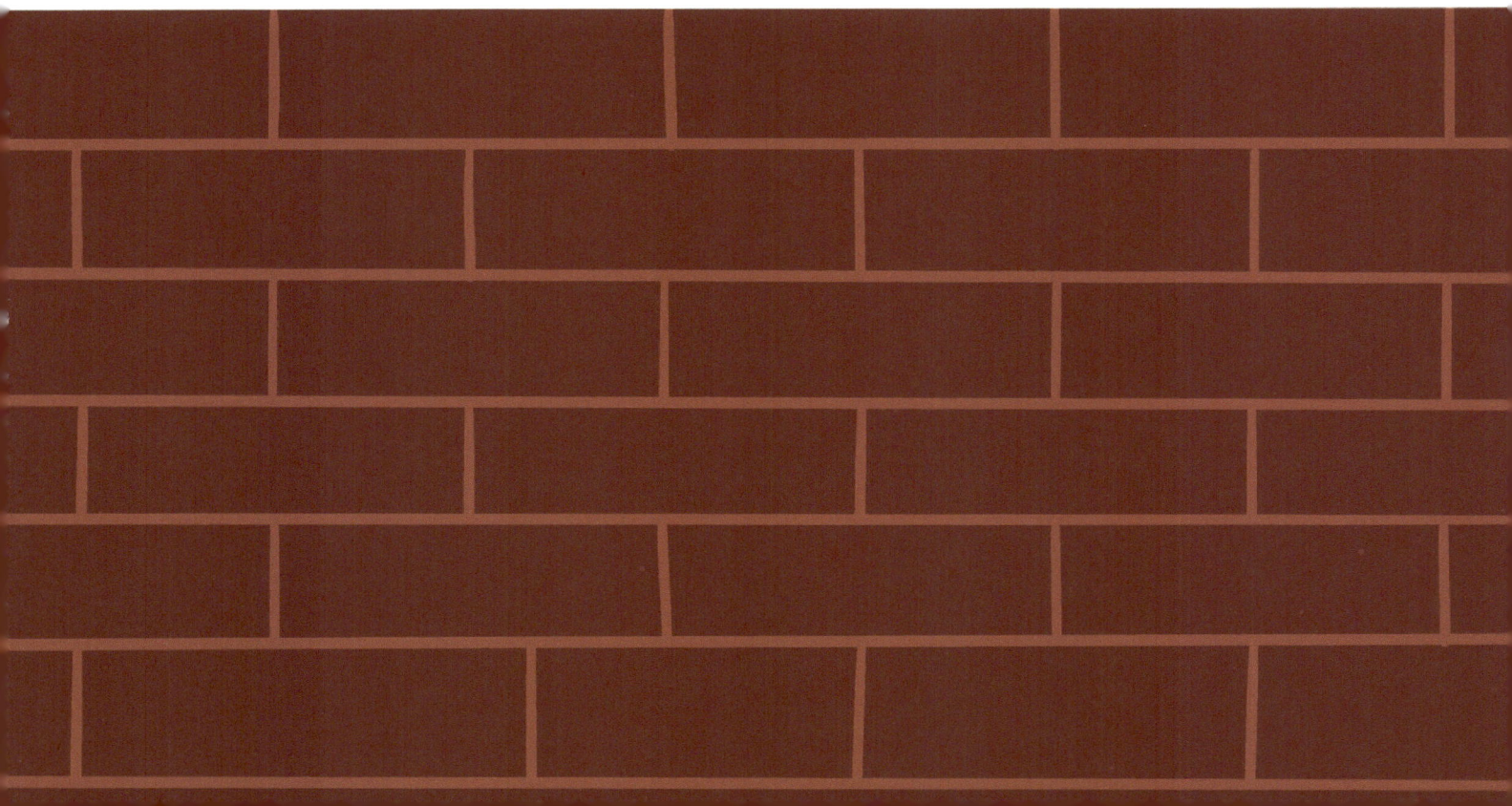

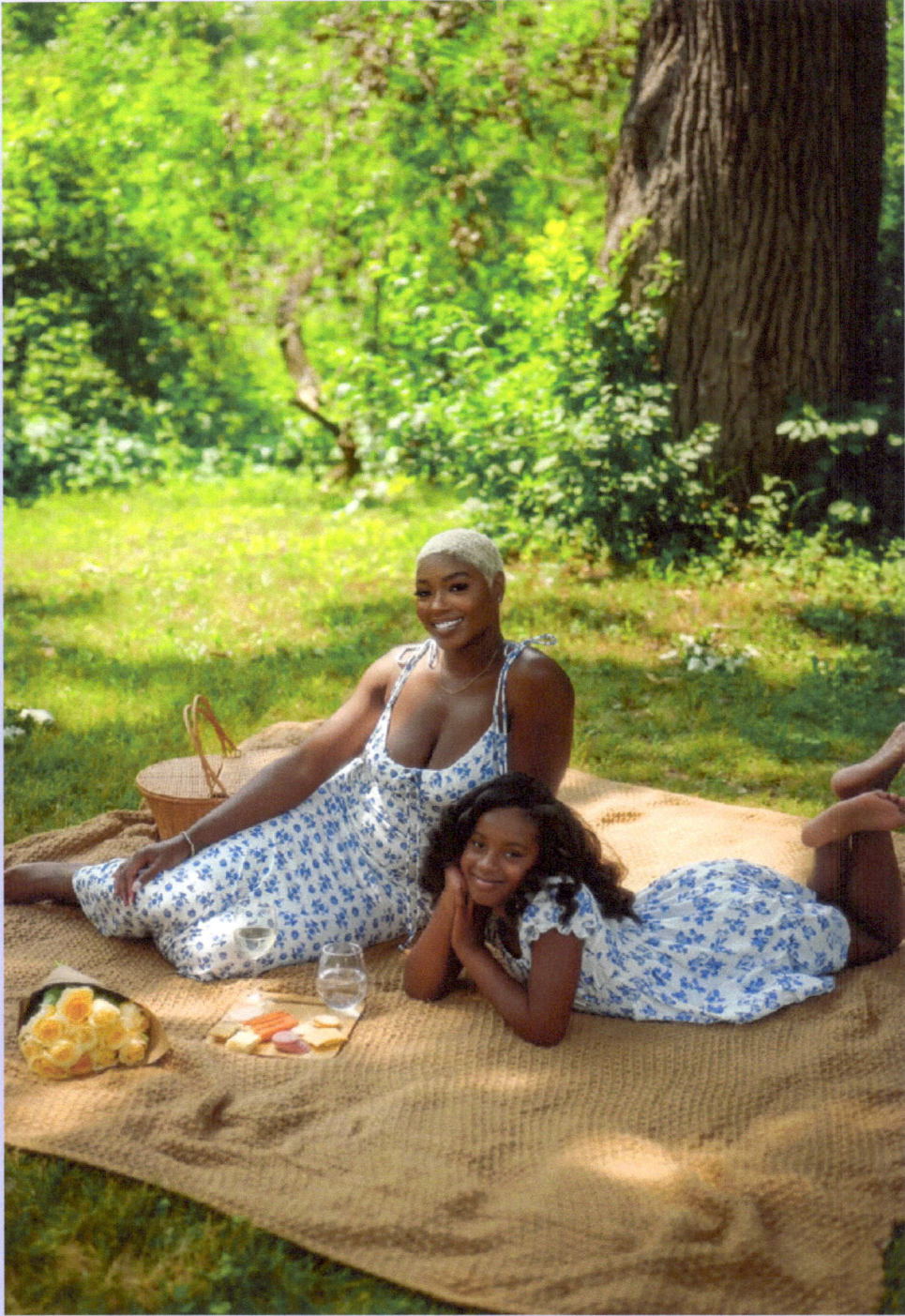

www.ingramcontent.com/pod-product-compliance
Lightning Source LLC
Chambersburg PA
CBHW041544260326
41914CB00015B/1538